Evolving the Dinosaur

REBUILDING PAEDIATRIC CLINICAL TRIALS AS A SERVICE

Violet Ford

EVOLVING THE DINOSAUR

Rebuilding Paediatric Clinical Trials as a Service

ISBN 978-1-5445-2023-0 *Hardcover*
978-1-5445-2022-3 *Paperback*
978-1-5445-2021-6 *Ebook*

LEVSHOW

DEDICATED TO MY PARENTS, WHO TAUGHT ME SELF-RELIANCE.

Contents

Terminology Used Interchangeably (or in Preference of)

Medicine, *medication*, and *drug* (in the context of a pharmaceutical substance used therapeutically) are used interchangeably throughout the book, even though there has been a move towards using the word *medicine* in preference of *drug*. Note the word *drug* has remained in *adverse drug reaction* (ADR).

Paediatric clinical research pharmacy, *pharmacy clinical trial service*, or *investigational drug service* are used interchangeably.

Paediatric pharmacy clinical trials/research as a service and *paediatric RaaS* or *pharmacy RaaS* or *RaaS* are used interchangeably.

Paediatric clinical trials and *paediatric investigational drug trials* and *investigational product trials* are used interchangeably.

Clinical trial pharmacists and *research pharmacists* are used in preference of *investigational drug pharmacists.*

Clinical research associate and *study monitor* are used interchangeably.

Clinical trial team, *research team*, and *site team* are used interchangeably.

Clinical trial visit, *clinical visit*, and *trial visit* are used interchangeably.

Clinical trial participant and *trial participant* and *research participant* are used interchangeably.

Investigational product and *investigational medicinal product* are used in preference of *investigational drug.*

Investigational products handling manual and *pharmacy manual* are used interchangeably.

Note: for this book, *pharmacovigilance* is used as defined by the World Health Organisation (WHO): 'The science and activities related to the detection, assessment, understanding and prevention of adverse drug effects or any other possible drug-related problems.' The scope of pharmacovigilance has grown remarkably. It includes ADRs or events, medication errors, counterfeit or substandard medicines, medicines misuse and/or abuse and interactions. Throughout paediatric trials implementation, pharmacists mainly survey medication errors, misuse, and assist principal investigators with reporting ADRs.

Abbreviations

ADME: Absorption, distribution, metabolism, and excretion

ADR: Adverse drug reaction

BW: Body weight

CRA: Clinical research associate

CRC: Clinical research coordinator

CRO: Contract research organisation (aka *clinical research organisation)*

CT: Clinical trials

CTA: Clinical trial agreement (otherwise known as *research agreement*)

CTMS: Clinical trial management system

EC: Ethics committee

FPFV: First patient's first visit date

FPLV: First patient's last visit date

GCP: Good clinical practice

GMP: Good manufacturing practice

GRP: Good research practice

IB: Investigator's brochure

ICH: International Conference on Harmonisation of Technical Requirements for Registration of Pharmaceuticals for Human Use

IM: Intramuscular

IMP: Investigational medicinal product

IP/ID: Investigational product/investigational drug

IPAL: Investigational product accountability log

IPHM: Investigational product handling manual (better known as pharmacy manual)

IRB: Institutional review board

IRT: Interactive response technology

IV: Intravenous

KPI: Key performance indicator

LPFV: Last patient's first visit date

LPLV: Last patient's last visit date

NG: Nasogastric

NTF: Note to file

PI: Principal investigator

PK: Pharmacokinetic

RaaS: Research as a service

SI: Sub investigator

SIV: Site initiation visit

SOP: Standard operational procedures

WFI: Water for injection

Introduction and Aim

'Sixty-five million years ago the dinosaurs had a bad day'.

—PHIL PLAIT

Kids love dinosaurs because they are big and powerful. Being extinct, they can be admired without the worry of bumping into one.

However, this book is not about dancing dinosaurs wishing sweet dreams to kids. Instead, it is about evolving a paediatric pharmacy managed clinical trials (CTs) service within the complex health system, where one solution cannot solve all problems, but small, safe, and high impact changes can drive faster transformation. *Evolving the Dinosaur* is a snapshot of how the service implemented a *change-measure-track* framework to attain higher performing systems that can support the increase in number and complexity of paediatric clinical trials to meet the needs and demands of the twenty-first century.

Evolving the Dinosaur represents intrapreneurship*; a stance for changing and adopting agile mindsets. This book was inspired by my passion for more effective and efficient trial services and enhanced participants experience.

We are accustomed to the Silicon Valley way of disrupting an industry from outside, disrupting quickly and dealing with consequences later. Unfortunately, the healthcare system cannot afford to 'move fast and break things.' It is evolving and advancing and cannot afford mistakes, even though it may need fast modernisation. While life-changing innovations in medical treatments are achieved at a reasonably rapid pace, improvements in healthcare delivery occur relatively slowly. The common denominator between the healthcare system, pharmacy profession, and paediatric research is that they are ethically challenging, heavily regulated, and not yet sufficiently standardised to enable rapid change.

Children have historically been excluded from clinical trials, but the landscape has changed after global legislative initiatives. Over the last twenty years, the science of paediatric drug development advanced and led to an increased number, variety, and complexity of CTs. To meet this exponentially increasing demand, hospitals' and health organisations' pharmacies began establishing specialised clinical trial services, a rapidly evolving area.

The answer to the question: What about the Dinosaur? Well, the Dinosaur's story is part of our own. They give us a real sense of the changes that can happen through time. If those champions of resilience and persistence continued to exist, they would have influenced mammalian evolution and had plenty of potential niches if not killed by an asteroid.

*Pharmacist intrapreneurs identify and pursue the implementation of new ideas into their area of practice. They make sacrifices and leverage existing knowledge, skills, and resources to implement changes or achieve the envisioned services or patient care improvements. The journey can be bumpy. We may not get a green light right away. We may experience initial rejection, setbacks, or have to work outside of our regular duties. The best advice is to keep our focus on the achievements, not on the hurdles.

WHAT TO EXPECT

This book is written by an intrapreneurial pharmacist who has made the journey. I assert that the variety of challenges and concerns tackled here are more than just CT pharmacists pain points. Many of them are consequences of substandard quality information resources, data collection tools, not well-thought-out safety initiatives, and IP packaging posing an increased risk of errors, all of which are provided to site pharmacies by sponsors or CROs. Understandably, external stakeholders cannot solve unknown problems.

The book is based on my personal experiences with data-driven change implementation over five years. I intend to show, rather than tell and humbly suggest, some feasible solutions, frameworks, tools for service improvements, practical how-tos, and tips and tricks for medicines administration in infants and children, which I have successfully used.

The framework and solutions stem from my twenty years of experience as an advanced paediatric pharmacist, an intrapreneur, and an expert in the field across global healthcare systems, industries, and academia. While it cannot be guaranteed that what worked incredibly well for me will work equally well for others, if considering implementing changes more effectively in a workplace, *Evolving the Dinosaur* will guide you to achieve desired results and create value-added services faster.

The book opens with brief information about the history of paediatric clinical research evolution and the key challenges. Then, it introduces site research team members, defines their roles and impact on each other, and recounts the interactions with pharmacy CT service.

Part 1 is dedicated to the journey of change management. It focuses on identifying services, processes, and workflows requiring change and implementing it with emphasis on what it takes and what to avoid, all while *Evolving the Dinosaur*. For example, building bridges with various stakeholders is crucial to avoid misunderstanding or resistance. Effective communication, active involvement, and radical collaboration, along with goals and resources alignment, are necessary for gaining stakeholders' engagement and commitment at each stage of a change management implementation.

Part 2 concentrates on measuring the implemented changes and the effectiveness of the framework. It also zeroes in on how to pre-select metrics to collect appropriate, accurate, and meaningful data, justified by examples. Finally, in Part 3, the focus is on the sustainability of the implemented change management through tracking the effectiveness of the service, workflows, and the performance of processes.

THE OBJECTIVES

DISSEMINATE AND ONBOARD KNOWLEDGE

The first objective of *Evolving the Dinosaur* is to disseminate and onboard knowledge, expertise, and experiences by attaining targeted and sustainable outcomes with the RaaS framework. I am not aware of any formal education or training program offered by institutions or universities on how to manage understaffed pharmacy CT/research service with an exponentially growing number of trials while also balancing participant safety, delivery of quality and value-added services, consumer satisfaction, *and* keeping up effective communication and collaboration with hundreds of internal and external research personnel simultaneously.

There are country-specific pharmacy guidelines for managing investigational products (IPs) and standards of practice in clinical trials, which pharmacists create, but their centre of attention is predominantly the pharmacists' duties. Books on paediatric drug development mostly focus on trial designs, challenges, stakeholder roles, ethical issues, regulatory changes, legislation, etcetera. Although these books offer a great deal of information and target a broad spectrum of readers, there is an awareness gap in the paediatric clinical research literature about the CT pharmacists, who manage the implementation of hundreds of trials simultaneously, despite protocols' complexity or the medication safety risks inherent to investigational product nomenclature, look alike, packaging, and unstandardised labelling.

I hope that by the end of the book, readers shift their perception of CT/research pharmacists from the health professionals who just dispense and perform IP accountability to the health professionals who—while managing the trial pharmaceuticals—are having multidimensional input into paediatric research.

Throughout trial execution, CT pharmacists encounter unique challenges to prevent and eliminate risks and errors and ensure participants' safety. Nevertheless, they remain unnoticed and under-consulted even on what is essential for them. Are pharmacists introverts who do not seek out attention? Are they research team misfits? Do they need to re-establish their professional identity and credibility in paediatric research? I hope to provide some answers to those intriguing questions.

Hospital pharmacy departments are restricted access areas. Thus, no internal health professionals or external parties, such as pharma industry representatives, sponsors, or members of the local research community, have direct access or detailed insights.

Hopefully, I shed some light and debunk the common belief that CT pharmacists have limited duties during trial implementation, only as specified by trial protocols.

RAISE AWARENESS OF MEDICATION SAFETY CONCERNS

The second objective of *Evolving the Dinosaur* is to raise awareness about medication safety concerns surrounding paediatric investigational products. Currently, an IP's error mitigation is managed mainly by the site's pharmacists. Unlike commercially available medications, there is limited regulatory guidance about their nomenclature, labelling, and packaging to promote safety. Although IP-related errors can affect data accuracy of safety and efficacy clinical trials, actual improvements are yet to be realised.

Similarly, IP handling manuals and accountability logs are not always aligned with safe paediatric practice, but these issues are not formally addressed as they do not require approval by ethics committees or institutional review boards (EC/IRBs).

INTRAPRENEURSHIP FOR YOUNG PHARMACISTS

The third objective of *Evolving the Dinosaur* is to advance the educational approach for the next generation of pharmacists considering clinical trials/research as a career. By introducing them to intrapreneurship in clinical trials and walking them step by step through the framework, they can master change management, achieve desired results and create value in their professional lives faster.

RaaS framework encourages pharmacists to get out of the department to organise participants' IP orders instead of waiting for them, to follow up on trial-related requirements, meet with research team members, and discuss streamlining cross-functional workflows. I found this approach very productive because it kept me well informed in advance of what, when, and why. My objective is to help others springboard faster by using the entire framework, or parts of it, subject to individual needs. The lessons learned and the benefits are itemised in the relevant chapters.

WHO WILL BENEFIT?

Evolving the Dinosaur is well-suited for people who are interested in the subject and read about it, for those who conduct paediatric clinical trials, and those directly or indirectly involved with clinical trials pharmacists.

Readers will gain a better understanding of the practice insights, challenges, and possible solutions that can improve quality IP-related information resources and the data collection tools to upsurge their accuracy. Furthermore, the proposed solutions can minimise safety risks and reduce senseless protocol deviations related to missing information or discrepancies between different resources.

Paediatric research stakeholders will gain more detailed insights into CT pharmacists' unique positioning and input, beyond IP handling, and catch on to why early and direct communication with them is crucial. Humble collaboration and working in synergy are fundamental to work out the best medication safety mitigation strategies.

Pharmacists will become more acquainted with identifying metrics, generating data, and implementing data-driven service improvements with a limited budget. In addition, they will gain confidence in what to measure to then translate it into a meaningful outcome and, finally, how to track the success of the implemented changes over time.

This book may not benefit individuals, who are:

- Not interested in developing an intrapreneurial mindset, in self-improvement, or workplace effectiveness.
- Not willing to try new things and embrace new opportunities.
- Satisfied with where they are, a service funding, or a lack of appropriately trained staff and time constraints are irrelevant.
- Working in inflexible workplaces with a rigid top-down chain of command, where changes can only happen after lengthy planning and projections, not by understanding of the immediate CT service needs.

THE AUTHOR

AN ADVANCED PAEDIATRIC PHARMACIST PRACTITIONER AND INTRAPRENEUR

By now, you may be asking: *Who is Violet Ford?* Or wondering what a pharmacist has to say about clinical trials when their role is not even defined in GCP. Principal investigators are entirely responsible for the research projects conduct at site level, including for the IPs.

My pharmacy degree was reinforced with a postgraduate diploma in clinical pharmacy at the Curtin University of Technology in Perth, Australia. My professional growth and experience span across various areas, from senior management and leadership to lecturing, teaching, mentoring, medication safety management, specialised clinical services, medicinal information, project management, and clinical trials/research.

I have spent nearly a decade at the front line of therapeutic care as critical care, renal, and cardiology pharmacist and a decade in the areas of paediatric medication safety, project management, and clinical trials. Altogether, I have been a practising pharmacist for four decades across global healthcare systems, industry, and academia.

I have dedicated the last twenty years to paediatrics and intrapreneurship. I have first-hand experience with the therapeutic challenges and the impact of the lack of evidence-based treatments and medicinal information for children.

Now, I am sharing my experience in establishing and implementing a framework for managing paediatric clinical trials/research as a service (RaaS) through data-driven changes, measurement, and tracking the outcomes. I am proud of the significant service, management, and cultural changes achieved throughout the framework implementation, resulting in high quality participants—centred services, increased safety, minimised number of IP errors, and protocol deviations contributing to completing the overall site's trials.

My passion for paediatric research and the logistics involved kept me attracted to this fascinating and challenging area. It does suit my personality because managing all aspects of a pharmacy CT service is not exactly written in books, and the area is fast-paced; the decision-making is facts-based and data-guided. Each new trial planning, set-up, and operational management presents different challenges, requiring different reasoning, problem-solving, professional and interpersonal skills to execute it most efficiently and cost-effectively while keeping participants' safety and their family's needs at the forefront.

ON THE FRONT LINE OF PAEDIATRIC CARE

Pharmacy is an old profession and has changed profoundly over the last forty years. I have had the opportunity to see its dynamic change, expansion, maturation, and increasing diversity. However, recently, I took a step aside in a pursuit to redirect my paediatric clinical knowledge and practice-derived expertise towards paediatric clinical trials solutions—advisory/consultancy and coaching services. So, I will briefly outline some of my professional endeavours to help you get to know me better.

I have had opportunities to join and work with great medical teams of different specialties as an advanced clinical pharmacist practitioner at Perth Children Hospital in Western Australia. Each specialty area had various but specific challenges. However, a few of them have had tremendous professional and personal impact and are the reason to embark on *Evolving the Dinosaur*.

Working as a paediatric critical care pharmacist was both challenging and rewarding. At the front line of therapeutic care, the environment is fast-paced, and the pressure is high because of the complex clinical enquiries and the need to make decisions on your feet. Daily, bedside patient rounds require going above and beyond to optimise treatments of the sickest patients in the hospital. However, the reward of becoming a specialised pharmacist and being an indispensable part of the hospital critical care multidisciplinary team was pleasing. The more years of experience I gained, the more patient care decisions I was entrusted to make. Working there reinforced my belief that miracles do happen.

While my first-hand experiences on the front line of paediatric care were challenging and rewarding, the inability to make informed medicinal/treatments decisions guided by adequate scientific evidence on doses, dosing, safety, and efficacy was quite frustrating.

THE MAIN IDEA

This book attempts to close the gap of the existing pharmacists' challenges throughout trials' implementation, their nature and root causes, and the unawareness of the problem to all other stakeholders involved.

I aspire to reinforce the urgency for more vital bridges between research pharmacists and drug development stakeholders and synergy in their quest to reduce or eliminate safety risks, improve information resources, participants experience, retention, and multidimensional compliance.

I intentionally provide an overview on how paediatric pharmacy CT service operations are managed manually, what the pharmacists' challenges and requirements are, and what they can bring to the table, as if not fully understood, they cannot be solved in the virtual space.

I have made the journey and now share my experience rebuilding paediatric pharmacy clinical trials/research as a service (RaaS) and the lessons learned during the change management and scaling the service up. The RaaS framework is practical and resulted in improved efficiency, quality trial management and services delivery. It is not based on a theoretical exploration of concepts but applied underpinnings. RaaS offers the infrastructure for managing the pharmaceutical part of clinical studies of different designs, types, and complexity.

PAEDIATRIC RAAS FRAMEWORK

The framework is participants-centred and has three main components: the change management journey, measurement plan, and tracking. It embraces scientific rigour and strict adherence to local legislation, the principles of Good Clinical Practice (GCP) and research protocol requirements. It is iterative. The strategies can be altered based on continuous monitoring feedback and repeated due to their solid foundation.

Change management encompasses identifying problems and possible solutions, assessing their impact on other stakeholders, pursuing their collaboration, and managing the obstacles during implementation. The measurement plan includes but is not limited to quantifying CT service operations, processes, and financials while keeping adherence to protocol, research and governance frameworks, and tracking to assess the success of the implemented changes.

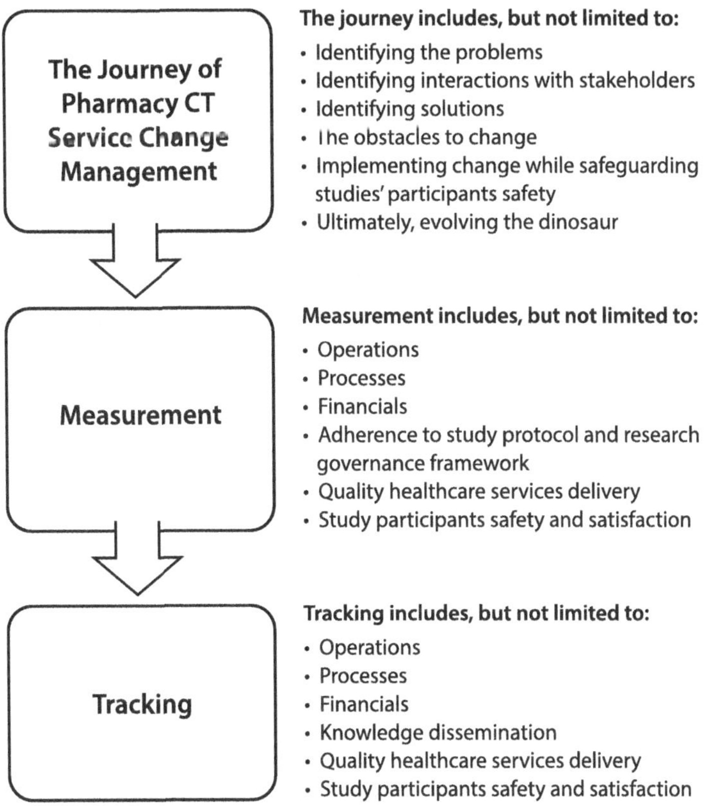

Fig. 1: A visual representation of Paediatric RaaS.

How did I embark on this journey? By setting a goal and establishing what should be measured and why; the purpose of each measurement. The goal was refined into several questions, which broke down the problem into its major components. Each question was then turned into a metric. Some metrics were used to answer different questions under the same goal. For example, the answers to general questions led to a general snapshot of the baseline service performance. Then, by digging deeper into individual processes and measuring their performance metrics, I identified specific ones needing improvement.

The critical point was to make sure that the questions I was trying to answer aligned with the problems I was solving and my goals. When the answer for both was yes, the collected answers led to a quality service improvement.

LESSONS LEARNED:

1. Data-guided solution implementation requires measurements of specific service or process performance metrics and then using the data to drive the best course of action.
2. Ongoing performance monitoring directs continual service improvements in the context of where we are, compared to where we intend to be, and enables us to make prompt adjustments.
3. Tracking metrics (such as participant safety, satisfaction, operational and financial performance, staff engagement, or the number of people leaving because of the implemented changes) closes the feedback loop on the effectiveness of the change management strategy and helps to identify if additional corrective actions are required.

Building/rebuilding pharmacy paediatric RaaS involves:

4. Purposeful change management that simultaneously improves quality services delivery and participants safety. This multistep journey encompasses identifying problems, monitoring interactions with stakeholders, noting the obstacles to change, and determining the best possible solutions and implementing them.

5. Measurement plan to quantify CT service operations, processes, financials, and adherence to protocol, research and governance framework.
6. Tracking the service operations, processes, financials, scope, and knowledge dissemination.

For accurate comparison over time and between entities, a defined start and endpoint and consistently using the same measuring units was crucial. The bottom line is that if we do not measure, we cannot improve. If we do not track, we cannot compare data trends or assess progress.

RAAS—CONTINUOUS IMPROVEMENTS

The ongoing improvements in pharmacy CT services were mainly focused on what mattered to the participants and the stakeholders involved. For example, streamlining dispensing and/or cross-functional clinical visits workflows improved efficiency, reduced/eliminated participants' waiting time for IP supply, and increased their satisfaction.

The RaaS framework was tested and refined over more than five years and across hundreds of CTs. It propelled the pharmacy CT service to evolve from traditional to data-driven. Additionally, it supported consistent improvements, focused on participants' safety, data integrity, greater compliance with GCP, trial protocol, relevant legislation, institutional research governance and ethics frameworks, and hospital and pharmacy policies and procedures.

This data-driven, bottom-up change management framework also transformed the service scope from basic clinical trials support to a more effective, efficient, and financially self-sustainable end-to-end trial service.

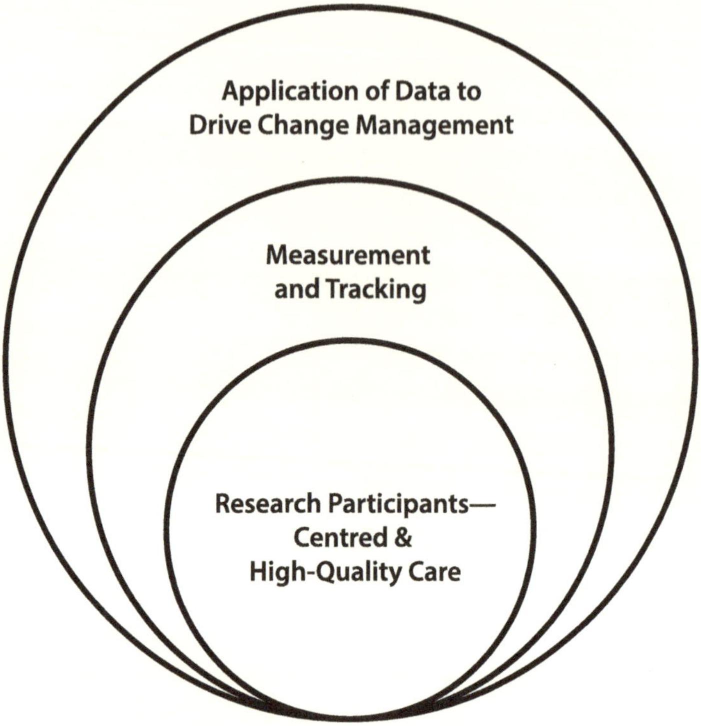

Fig. 2: A visual representation of the participant centred RaaS.

CONTEMPORARY CLINICAL TRIAL/RESEARCH PHARMACY PRACTICE

A clinical trials/research pharmacist is a unique and exciting job and is theoretically well known, but it is not. I have been genuinely questioned by other researchers, external stakeholders, and even colleague pharmacists about what I do, apart from IP management and dispensing. It appeared that in clinical research, pharmacists remain the invisible health professionals to the outside world, irrespective of the various hurdles they must overcome to improve their services and efficiency to improve participants' safety and data integrity within exceedingly complex trial protocols requirements.

CT pharmacists carry the responsibility to continually improve their effectiveness and value-added services so as to accommodate the increased demand for paediatric pharmacy trial services in parallel with the exponential growth in number, variety, and complexity.

I am proud of the significant changes implemented between January 2014 and May 2019 at Westhead Children's Hospital in Sydney. Maybe not all those changes will survive past my leaving the role or be kept active, but I am pretty pleased with the successful results in *Evolving the Dinosaur.*

No one decides to explore what can be changed at work or suddenly notices the top-down decision-making barriers that affect the quality or effectiveness of the services they are providing. Do we choose to make bottom-up changes because it is a good idea? Both management styles, top-down and bottom-up, have pros and cons, so how do we assess which one is better for our circumstances? Whose support will be required? What effective method will be employed? Who will be affected? What is the goal? Moreover, how will it be executed?

The answers to those questions and how further evolve pharmacy clinical trials within a complex healthcare system, where different solutions have their tools and logic, are outlined throughout the book.

In healthcare, one size does not fit all solutions, but small, high impact changes can improve efficiencies, effectiveness, and accelerate changes.

Evolving the Dinosaur is about applying new frameworks, rebuilding an existing paediatric CT service, and implementing change-measure-track loops to attain high performing systems to meet the increased demands for high quality paediatric research.

PART ONE

The Change Management Journey of *Evolving the Dinosaur*

'Management is about persuading people to do things they do not want to do, while leadership is about inspiring people to do things, they never thought they could'.

—STEVE JOBS

CHAPTER ONE

Paediatric Clinical Trials

'Continuous improvement is better than delayed perfection'.

—MARK TWAIN

WHY PAEDIATRIC RESEARCH IS IMPORTANT

Most of the currently registered medicines traditionally have been developed, studied, and approved for use in the adult population, thus lacking evidence of proven safety, efficacy, and dosing for paediatric patients. Presently, more than 50 per cent of all medicines prescribed to children do not have adequate label information, and more than 90 per cent have not been studied in neonates.

Pharmaceutical therapy in paediatric clinical practice continues to be supported by low-quality safety and efficacy evidence. It is mainly guided by the physicians' personal experience and their moral intention to treat infants and children with off-label medicines, unapproved for the age group or indications or dosage or route of administration.

Paediatric clinical trials are performed in children and adolescents under eighteen years of age to assess the safety and effectiveness of new medicinal products for claimed indications and establish safe and effective dosing for administration in the different age subpopulations. An investigational product is considered new, even if it has been used for years, when presented in a new formulation or dosing regimen, proposed for a different route of administration, or used in a different patient's population, posing an increased risk.

Paediatric drug development is fundamental to ensure infants and children have access to high quality, age appropriate, reliably evaluated, and evidence-based pharmaceutical formulations for paediatric diseases, which are a substantial public health burden and a concern. Clinical trials are a core step in a new drug development process. Through them, the clinical, pharmacological, and pharmacodynamic aspects of investigational products are established.

The stages of the drug development process are as follows:

Stage 1: Discovery and Development →
Stage 2: Preclinical →
Stage 3: Clinical Trials →
Stage 4: Regulatory Application →
Stage 5: Approval

During the *discovery stage*, a promising compound for development is identified.

Throughout the *development stage*, further experiments are conducted to collect information about absorption, distribution, metabolism, excretion, potential benefits, mechanisms of action, appropriate dosage form (tablet, injection, etc.), adverse events, interactions with other medicines, and treatments and effectiveness in comparison to other similar medicinal products.

The *preclinical studies* stage provides information on dosing and toxicity. If the results are positive, the new investigational product(s) can be tested in people through clinical trials to evaluate their safety and efficacy and satisfy all requirements for regulatory approval.

To sum up, paediatric drug development is essential to ensure children have access to high quality healthcare, similar to adults, with reliably evaluated and evidence-based age-appropriate pharmaceutical formulations. In addition, pharmaceutical therapy for paediatric patients must be guided by adequate scientific evidence about medicinal dose/dosing, safety, and efficacy to allow physicians to make informed decisions for their patients.

THERAPEUTIC ORPHANS? WHAT CHANGED THE LANDSCAPE?

More than fifty years ago (in 1968), Dr H. Shirkey addressed infants and children as 'therapeutic or pharmaceutical orphans.' Historically, drug law changes (in 1938 and 1962) came to pass only after paediatric tragedies, such as deaths from sulfanilamide elixir, which contained diethylene glycol, a toxic excipient, and congenital disabilities (phocomelia) due to maternal exposure to thalidomide during pregnancy.[1] As a result, many medicines released after that carried a clause 'not to be used in infants and children' or 'not recommended' due to a lack of clinical data to establish recommendations for safe use in paediatric patients.

Legislative changes led to the adoption of the therapeutic orphans and a boom in paediatric clinical trials.

More than twenty-five years later, in 1994, the Pediatric Pharmacology Research Unit (PPRU) Network was created to support pharmaceutical testing in children. Since then, federal laws and regulations were introduced and adopted, which led to an increased number and variety of paediatric clinical trials and an increased number of medicines labelled for use in children. In addition, different incentives, such as the paediatric exclusivity provision, which granted extended patent protection or market exclusivity to manufacturers conducting voluntary CTs of new drugs in children, have encouraged paediatric research growth.

To promote and support the development of new medicines for paediatric use, the US Congress passed the Pediatric Research Equity Act (PREA) and Best Pharmaceuticals for Children Act (BPCA). The US laws and regulations inspired the European Union, and in 2007, the current EU Paediatric Regulation was embraced. By offering some valuable incentives, pharmaceutical companies are required to perform paediatric CTs essential to providing safe and effective healthcare for children.

The legislative incentives, coupled with the increased pharmaceutical industry commitment, led to an increased interest in paediatric drug research, resulting in a significantly higher number and variety of clinical trials with increased complexity.

THE CHALLENGES

Why discuss the challenges in paediatric clinical trials? Because the evolution of paediatric research encouraged additional paediatric clinical trials. However, their challenges remain unchanged. Children are entitled to the same level of pharmaceutical treatment standards as adults. If the challenges cannot be avoided, *building foundations and dedicating additional resources towards conducting higher-level paediatric research may be the way forward.* I will provide an introductory overview of the most crucial challenges, as they are outside the scope of this book.

The main challenges for the pharmaceutical industry are high development costs and limited financial gain. Drug development is generally a highly regulated process designed to ensure the safest and most effective drugs reach the market for individual use. Extra toxicity tests are required for the paediatric population, including the additional cost for developing age-appropriate formulations. It takes around ten years and an average estimated cost above $2.6 billion to bring a new medicine to market.

Paediatric drug development is difficult and complex due to the influence of children's age, growth, biological and physiological functions development, and the effect of disease states on the investigational drugs' pharmacokinetic (PK) parameters—absorption, distribution, metabolism, and excretion (ADME)—which are altered to varying degrees during the developmental stages.

The paediatric population is diverse, with different physiologies across different age subgroups:

- Preterm neonates: less than thirty-six weeks
- Full term neonates: birth to thirty days
- Infants: one month to one year
- Toddlers: one to four years
- Children: five to twelve years
- Adolescents: twelve to eighteen years

The paediatric population's major organs and body systems mature in size and function during infancy and childhood at different rates; thus, drug dose-response and adverse reactions vary during childhood. Proportions of body fat, protein, and extracellular water change continuously during infancy and childhood, affecting dose sizes per kilogram of body weight. Oral absorption is affected by developmental changes in the gastrointestinal tract. Gastric acidity, intestinal pH, emptying time, gut motility, and surface area vary in different age subgroups.

Pharmacodynamic differences are due to target receptors', transporters', and channels' developmental processes.[2] For example, morphine-related respiratory depression and bradycardia in neonates are due to underdevelopment of opioid receptors.

CENTRAL CHALLENGES:

- Paediatric trial designs require a solid foundation, analytical thinking, a high level of awareness, and consideration of various possible risks and factors that may affect trial conduct and successful completion.
- Finding adequately trained *paediatric investigators with institutional infrastructure and support.* CT implementation on a site level is a multidisciplinary effort; thus, the availability of dedicated and appropriately trained research coordinators and pharmacists is equally essential.
- Recruitment difficulties are mainly related to the limited number of eligible patients with a specific disease.
- CTs' inclusion and exclusion criteria can be highly restrictive, negatively affecting recruitment.
- The small number of participants with a particular disease may affect the ability to establish study treatment outcomes.

- Pharmacokinetic and pharmacodynamic studies may require different formulations.
- Lack of correlation between safety, pharmacokinetic, and pharmacodynamic parameters between adults and children makes it difficult to establish how those parameters differ in children.
- Age-appropriate formulations with more straightforward dosing schedules, while positively influence participants' IP compliance, are hard to achieve.
- Paediatric CTs require establishing safety and efficacy for different age groups because of the age-related altered pharmacokinetic parameters at various developmental stages.

Further, there are ethical issues with parents/guardians consenting to their child's participation in clinical trials due to children's inability to understand or assess potential risks fully. Participant's enrolment/retention difficulties may arise with children ages seven or older because they can assent or dissent to their participation in a trial.

Likewise, there are ethical concerns about the inclusion of children in clinical trials and about the research questions or the design, including the uncertainty of the new treatment success versus the fear of willingly exposing a child to an unproven therapy that may end up ineffective or more harmful than an existing standard treatment.

As challenging as they are, paediatric trial designs should not have room for the potential to harm by disregarding children's specific issues. Therefore, a comprehensive provision of a systematic literature review justifying the trial, the impact of the disease, age and development-specific outcomes, a statistical analysis plan, and specified intention to treat analysis are imperative.

Paediatric formulations are difficult to develop, owing to numerous considerations, such as chemical and physical characteristics of active ingredient(s), choice of excipients to avoid possible adverse reactions, age-appropriate formulations with further attention to the taste, smell, and volume per dose, to name a few. Furthermore, the IP form's appropriateness for accurate dosing and administration at home is crucial because medication adherence is achieved by focussing on participants and their parents or caregivers.

In summary, paediatric formulations are challenging from a technical point of view. They are more time consuming to make, are extra costly, and pose increased safety and liability risks.

Paediatric trial designs require a solid foundation and awareness of possible risks and implementation difficulties. Factors that can affect participants retention are the number, duration and frequency of clinical visits, the number of invasive or painful procedures, IP dosing frequency, and trial duration.

Stakeholders involved in clinical trial design, review, and approval carry an enormous obligation to ensure measures and outcomes are age-appropriate and that patients' health-related quality of life is taken under consideration. Nevertheless, successful CTs completion gets children a step closer to having access to a similar level and standard of healthcare as adults.

DO SOME PAEDIATRIC CLINICAL TRIALS FAIL?

The topic of failed paediatric clinical trials and the common contributing factors is vital for future improvements, but it is not within the scope of this book. Thus, intentionally, I am presenting brief statistical information and some critical reasons for general information. Research informs that up to 42 per cent of recently completed paediatric clinical trials have failed to establish either safety or efficacy, leading to the inability to label those products for use in children.[3] Knowing the causative factors is essential for better future design and formulating appropriate solutions to decrease the failure rate. Major contributing factors identified from publicly available FDA labels, medical, statistical, and clinical pharmacology reviews are:

- Inappropriate dose selection
- Clinical trial design
- Differences between paediatric and adult disease processes
- Higher placebo response in children

Inappropriate dose selection is a well-documented cause for paediatric trials' failures. For example, using dose escalation to determine the maximum tolerated dose may not establish efficacy. If no dosage range is studied, the tested dose may fail to demonstrate efficacy. Another example is when a dose selection is based on adults' lower end dose. Identifying the optimal paediatric dose is fundamental. Testing dose ranges is more helpful for defining dose-response relationships; however, it may not always be feasible, especially in trials for rare diseases, where the number of eligible participants is limited.

CT design was identified as a potential contributing factor in 30 per cent of the paediatric CTs submitted to the FDA between 2007 and 2014 but failed to establish a new or expanded paediatric indication. As outlined by Momper et al., inadequate design can be due to lack of an active comparator group, failure to consider the differences of disease mechanisms in children compared to adults, poor assay sensitivity, and the exclusion of placebo responders.

These examples highlight the requirement for tailoring paediatric study designs, to deliver a meaningful and interpretable outcome.[4]

Following a comprehensive assessment of the scientific and ethical implications, a sound choice of active comparator therapy selection would be the best available treatment to ensure children are exposed to current best available therapies.[5] Review by the European Medicine Agency in 2013 indicated problematic justifications of comparator selections in 28 per cent of the paediatric CTs.[6] The comparator choice should be made by using the most appropriate, paediatric-specific, evidence-based guidelines.

A lack of an appropriately documented dosing history, such as dose size, dosing time, or infusion rate, may affect or prevent correctly establishing a time/plasma concentrations course during trial implementation.

Another identified potential contributor to trials failure is the inter-subjects' pharmacokinetic variability in children, which, in some cases, can be substantially higher than in adults.[7]

High placebo response in paediatric patients has been recognised as an additional contributing factor for clinical trials' failure. K. Weimer et al. (2013) reviewed the placebo effect and its causes in paediatric patients and concluded that the placebo effect correlates negatively to age. The current research findings of substantial placebo response in children warrant attention when 'extrapolating drug efficacy in children from respective studies in adults runs the risk of underestimating the placebo response and overestimating drug efficacy'. Also, when relevant, consideration may be given to trial designs to include placebo run-in phases to reduce its effect on trial results.[8]

The consequences of paediatric CTs' failures are substantial: delays in label approvals, delayed access to appropriately evaluated medicines, continued use of off-label or unlicensed medicines instead of safe and effective, evidence-based therapies, and substantial financial setbacks for the pharmaceutical industry.

Unquestionably, trial design optimisation requires close stakeholders' collaboration and early engagement with regulatory authorities and experts in the field, including paediatric pharmacists, to actively contribute towards the final goal of timely approval of new, innovative, and safe medications for children.

One noteworthy point is the importance of publishing and sharing the results of completed CTs with the paediatric research community. For example, over the course of three years (2008 to 2011), Harvard University researchers reviewed more than 550 US federal government registered paediatric trials and found that more than 40 per cent were never completed. Furthermore, those that were completed were never published. Since then, publications-related regulatory measures have been applied to improve paediatric research outcomes sharing.

WHAT IT IS LIKE TO WORK WHILE *EVOLVING THE DINOSAUR*

'Intrapreneurship is an attitude, not a department'.

—DAWN ELIZABETH

Evolving the Dinosaur through intrapreneurial instigated initiatives within the healthcare system requires overcoming various hurdles. Initiatives can be rejected or discouraged, requiring outmanoeuvring a few administrators on the way to bring the ideas to life. At times, it feels like swimming against the stream.

Often you are on your own against outdated strategies in a system of multilayered management and bureaucracy, where it takes ages to get things done. The rigid hierarchy between professions (within professions and between organisational positions) inherent to public health organisations does not encourage employees to feel they are expected to take initiative, but to follow the rules. It can be discouraging and requires self-motivation and maintaining a positive spirit to move forward. Healthcare practitioners pursue and implement changes regardless of the challenges.

An individual intrapreneurship within a public hospital positively impacts *Evolving the Dinosaur*, even though it may require crossing existing boundaries, decentralising decision-making power based on expertise, not on position, and building bridges with various stakeholders to gain their engagement and commitment. Effective communication, consultations, active involvement, and radical collaboration to align goals and resources are crucial for the final success.

Health organisations are full of clinical staff with intrapreneurial mindsets. Irrespective of their background, level of expertise, or medical specialty, staff are supportive, accommodating, and helpful throughout the change implementation, particularly when the changes are targeted to improve healthcare services delivery and patients' care. For example, while an administrator may insist that all patients must wait for their medicine(s) supply because public hospitals cannot offer priority or expedited services, a senior medical practitioner does not mind walking to the pharmacy to hand in a prescription in-person, to speed up a patient's discharge. My way of thanking trial participants for tolerating the long and exhausting clinical visits was to have their IPs dispensed and ready before the end of the visit, thus eliminating waiting time for pharmacy services.

The World Health Organisation (WHO) has identified that patient waiting time for healthcare services is one of the critical measurements of a responsive health system. Likewise, long waiting times for IP supplies is disadvantageous for participants and their parents. Disadvantage inevitably leads to dissatisfaction. Indeed, it is challenging to retain dissatisfied participants in clinical trials. Is there a solution? Yes! We can reduce waiting time, increase our value-added services, expand participants' and parents' satisfaction, and improve the site CT teams' emotional fulfilment by instigating change management, more effective collaboration with PIs/trials team members/other stakeholders and streamlining workflows.

PHARMACY CLINICAL TRIALS/RESEARCH SERVICE

Paediatric pharmacy managed CT services are a specialised area that provides support and guidance for the safe and efficient conduct of clinical trials. They operate under different models, depending on the hospital type, research volume, pharmacy staff expertise, scope of services provided, and location of operation—from inside or outside the pharmacy department.

STAFFING MODELS

Depending on the institutional type, clinical research structure, volume, and complexity, clinical trial areas may be managed by a full time or a part-time pharmacist, a dedicated research pharmacist, or a team of specialised pharmacists and technicians.

FUNDING MODELS

Pharmacy CT services may operate on direct cost recovery from sponsors, indirectly funded by institutional grants to conduct research, through institutional funding for performed CTs, or the institution absorbs the clinical research costs.

WHO PROVIDES THE SERVICES?

Hospitals and healthcare services are the leading centres for clinical trials implementation. Consequently, the pharmacists in these institutions are directly involved, utilising their professional expertise, GCP and pharmacy best practices principles.

As qualified medicines experts, pharmacists are best suited to take on investigational products management to ensure safe and ethical use, handling, appropriate storage, and safe disposal. Furthermore, during trial implementation, their practices are aligned with continuous improvement of participant safety, protecting data integrity, and maintaining compliance with the approved research protocol and applicable regulations, including the International Conference on Harmonisation of Technical Requirements for Registration of Pharmaceuticals for Human Use (ICH) E6(R2) GCP and good manufacturing practice (GMP).

THE CLINICAL TRIAL TEAM

Who are the clinical trial team members? What are their duties, relations, and impact on each other?

Commonly, site clinical trial teams include:

- Principal investigator (PI) and sub investigator(s) SI(s)

- Clinical research coordinators (CRCs)
- Lead or senior CT/research pharmacist(s)
- Other pharmacists and pharmacy support staff (appropriately trained in all or specific CTs)

Other stakeholders working closely with the site during the implementation are:

- Sponsor or their delegates
- Contracted research organisation (CRO) representatives
- CT site monitors, also known as clinical research associates (CRAs)

MULTIFACETED CROSS-FUNCTIONAL RELATIONSHIPS

PRINCIPAL INVESTIGATORS (PI)

PIs are responsible for the conduct of clinical research projects at a site level, including IP accountability, storage, and use as per approved protocols. They delegate IP management to the pharmacy, but the delicate part is that PIs are not in charge of pharmacists, nor do they manage their professional practice and legal responsibilities under applicable laws, standards, and pharmacy or hospital guidelines. PIs do not have a managerial overlook over the CT service or pharmacy staffing; thus, they may not even be aware of inadequate human or equipment recourses. Pharmacy senior management oversees the departmental human resources, operations, clinical programs, informatics, and customer service. However, they may not be versed in the actual CT service performance or capacity status or know the number of active trials managed at any given time or their complexity, or current and future resources requirements. In the absence of reliable data, the decision making tends to be driven by conformational yeses to each new research project.

But can such practice support quality services? Can new clinical trials just be fit in between other pharmacy services?

Yes, for the basic CT service scope. No, for participant-centred services and of end to end scope of service. The consequences of pharmacy overcommitment will be discussed later. The point is that pharmacy CT services can move towards data-driven management and decision making to meet the increased demand for paediatric trials. Collecting and analysing quality data on service operational and financial performance, research volume and complexity, and participant experiences can drive targeted changes.

To better support institutional PIs and new paediatric research projects, the pharmacy CT services must adopt data-guided decision making instead of good intentions driven decision making.

CLINICAL TRIALS / RESEARCH PHARMACISTS

CT pharmacists have very unusual positioning within the research space. Their roles can vary to suit the organisation and pharmacy clinical needs. Pharmacists' duty of care encompasses much more than identifying and rectifying prescribing or dispensing errors. They are expected to recognise potential risks and intervene to prevent harm to patients by exercising professional judgement and discretion. However, in clinical research, their discernibility is not comparable to other team members, who may or may not even be health professionals and similarly perform only delegated tasks. This gap in responsibilities versus visibility is not explored, documented, or addressed formally.

Legally and professionally, pharmacists carry actual accountability over registered medicines and investigational products management, but in clinical research, it is a delegated responsibility. Maybe they should be independent team member.

As medical professionals, it seems more appropriate that PIs are responsible for trial conduct and participant management while CT pharmacists, as a separate entity, are independently in charge of the study pharmaceuticals and communicate/deal directly with sponsors or their delegates. It may take years before we see such changes.

PHARMACISTS VS OTHER CLINICAL TRIAL STAKEHOLDERS

Pharmacists are required to complete GCP training, and by doing so, they become aware of the roles, responsibilities, and obligations of sponsors, PIs, CROs, monitors and auditors. What other stakeholders know about the CT pharmacy services? Where can they find information? Currently their awareness is restricted to the tasks outlined in study protocols and pharmacy manuals.

Historically, pharmacists have earned their place inside the pharmacy, dispensing medicines, even though their scope of *practice* has *changed* substantially over the years. In clinical trials, it appears they are expected to do what they have always done, which limits their ability to collaborate, to meet other research stakeholders, or to participate in team meetings or discussions. The net result can be an actual or perceived feeling of being a misfit, working in isolation.

It has been noted that very few research stakeholders are familiar with the complexities and intricacies inherent to the CT pharmacists' practice. During a new budget negotiation, the pharmacy fees are frequently negotiated over more extended periods than they should be, due to the same reasons: a gap in awareness about pharmacy budget components and how they are calculated. The established perception that pharmacists just hand out IPs to trial participants cannot be changed rapidly.

This book provides insightful information intended to enhance readers understanding of how to better align their goals with site CT pharmacists, in addition to the traditional interactions with the PIs and research coordinators. Paediatric clinical trials cannot be fully understood if all stakeholders' contributions are not considered together as a whole. Successful completion does not belong to one specific individual or group, but rather to everyone involved and relies on their expertise, input, and collaboration.

Next, I will reflect on site team interactions and roles, outline their awareness of each other's input (or the lack thereof), and the effect of non-inclusion of CT pharmacists in new trial decision making.

CLINICAL RESEARCH CENTRE

Teaching hospitals may have a dedicated clinical research centre to facilitate research operational activities of industry-sponsored and investigator-initiated research. In addition, they may provide technical support, such as statistical analysis and administrative support, by providing research assistants and coordinators. They may also provide facility support in terms of information technology and workstations and conduct courses such as GCP, good research practice (GRP), and research methodology and biostatistics, including regular in house continuous professional development sessions on research methodology, study design, protocol development, and statistical analysis. Keeping in mind what functions the site's research centres have, it is apparent that CT/research pharmacists need to maintain regular communication, interactions, and radical collaboration to achieve complete inclusion in each step of new CT decision making.

INCLUSION/NON-INCLUSION IN A NEW CLINICAL TRIAL: PROS AND CONS

A new clinical trial at the site level usually starts with a feasibility assessment visit. Then, if the site is selected to conduct the trial, the following steps are preparing a budget, site initiation visit, trial implementation, and the final step is a closeout visit. These steps are thoroughly examined and discussed in Chapter 6, under the heading: 'New Clinical Trials', but here the focus is on the benefits and disadvantages of pharmacists' non-inclusion in each one.

SITE FEASIBILITY OR QUALIFICATION VISIT

The *feasibility assessmen*t is the process of evaluating the possibility of conducting a specific research project against the site's and pharmacy CT service's capability to fulfil its requirements.

During those visits, the sponsor or delegate presents the new trial protocol and inspects the site facility, equipment, policies, procedures, and other requirements. CT pharmacists must attend and collect necessary information to determine their own capacity to support the proposed trial.

Initial non-inclusion of pharmacists' is an ineffective practice in the long run and can lead to numerous negative consequences, such as:

- Project commencements delay due to limited time for pre-planning and organising required resources, including coordinating pharmacy matters to meet trial demands.
- Overburdening CT pharmacists lead to enormous pressure and distress, resulting in staff turnover, which can cause further delays.
- Rushed pharmacy trial-related setup may result in creating substandard dispensing summaries, unsafe practices, errors on accountability log entries, and omissions of dispensing steps (such as weighting IP bottles), affecting the establishment of accurate participant medication compliance.

The practice or established culture of non-inclusion of supporting departments representatives, including pharmacists, into the decision-making process during the initial evaluations of site capability does not support efficiency, safety or team cohesion, seamless workflows, and participants journeys.

I will briefly touch on the reasons for pharmacists' non-inclusion.

There is a vast interinstitutional and inter-PIs variation in research operational practices and deciding which new CTs will be taken on board and when to involve other supporting departments. For example, some PIs prefer to consult the team members ahead of time, while others decide by themselves and omit consultations/discussions, knowing they carry full responsibility for a CT's administration and ask for support later. Their attitudes may be influenced by previous experiences, CT pharmacist's credibility, effectiveness, helpfulness, and operational performance.

The main reasons for omitting early pharmacy involvement are the following:

First, limited awareness of the pharmacy CT service scope of involvement and operational practice, and second, the PIs primarily focus on the new trial scientific merits. Particularly if the institutional new research project approval process does not require written pharmacy authorisation or mandate CT pharmacists' early input.

PIs conducting multiple trials with multiple sponsors may decide in a silo which research projects to take on. They may complete site feasibility questionnaires and tick the boxes without considering the impact on supporting departments, driven by the fallacy of presumption that if it was all right in the past, it should be fine presently, too. However, as mentioned elsewhere in the book, a successful CT completion does not belong to one specific individual or group functioning in silos, but rather to everyone involved, relying on their expertise, input, and collaboration.

PHARMACY BUDGET

Depending on the pharmacy CT service funding model and the institutional research operational practice, the fees for the pharmaceutical portion of a clinical trial are either prepared by pharmacists, PIs, or an institutional research centre, using pre-determined pharmacy fees across all trials or fees previously provided for other projects. The advantages of applying the exact fees are mainly convenience and streamlining. The disadvantages are under-or over-budgeting depending on the trial's complexity, the number of participants to be enrolled, protocol requirements, and duration. However, the most crucial disadvantage is that CT pharmacists preapprove their exclusion from the budgeting step.

SITE INITIATION VISIT (SIV)

An SIV is a monitoring visit before the start of a trial. Its purpose is to ensure that the site is ready to enroll participants. Also, during the visit, the protocol is discussed, all queries answered, the trial team members are trained, and all precautions are taken to avoid unnecessary setbacks. Keeping in mind the SIV's purpose, it is expected that CT pharmacists are fully included in the protocol presentation and not only to cover the pharmacy materials. Such brief contact between pharmacy and sponsor or their delegate is neither full inclusion nor appropriate training for pharmacy staff.

CLINICAL TRIAL IMPLEMENTATION

CT pharmacists are always included. It is an obligation-driven inclusion for management of the investigational products, as per study protocol.

MONITORING VISITS

The purpose of the site monitoring visits is to review the trial's progress and ensure protocol adherence, data accuracy, participant safety, compliance with regulatory requirements, and good clinical practice guidelines (GCP).

CT pharmacists are included because the trial monitor must reconcile IPs and verify that appropriate storage has been maintained. While PI's and CRC's availability takes priority, confirmed monitoring visits without an appointment with a CT pharmacist are counterproductive, due to pharmacists' time constraints, clashes with other monitoring visits, lack of working space, and maintaining trial records confidentiality.

CLINICAL TRIAL CLOSE OUT VISIT

Usually, by the end of the trial, cross-functional relations are established, and monitors organise the close out visit directly with CT pharmacists.

Next, I will explore what impact, if any, the inclusion/non-inclusion of CT pharmacists might have on trial conduct. When not included in all steps, pharmacists are neither totally included nor excluded. Even omitted from a single step may lead to setbacks, due to unanticipated issues with meeting demands on short notice.

If inclusion/non-inclusion is depicted as a continuum, the closer to totally non-included pharmacists are, the greater their perceived feelings are of being a team misfit, leading to tension in team functionality with eventual impact on quality services.

What would it be like if CT pharmacists are fully included? A visual representation of the proposed CT pharmacist inclusion model is shown in Figure 3.

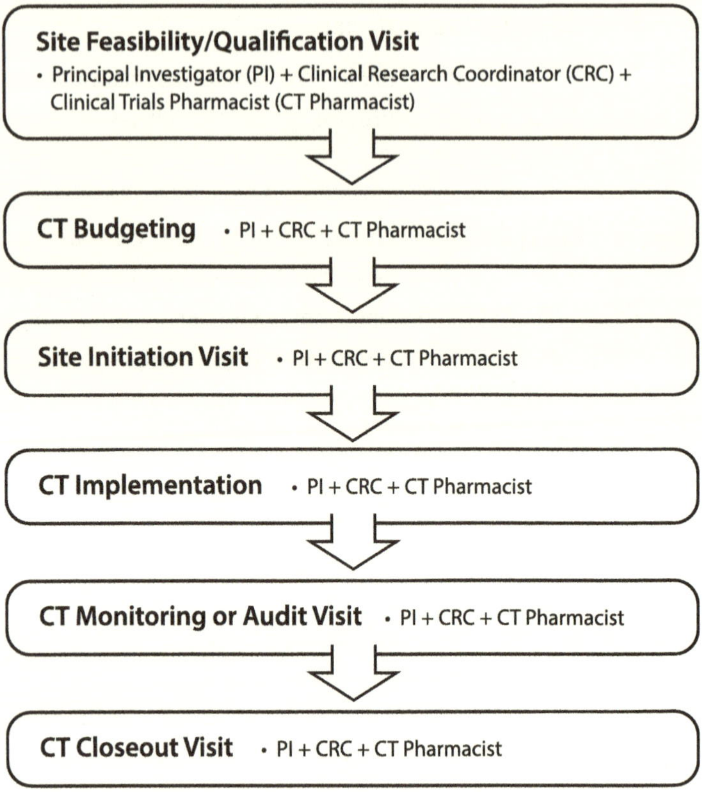

Fig. 3: Proposed CT pharmacist inclusion model in paediatric trials.

CHAPTER TWO

Paediatric Clinical Trial Pharmacists

HOW DO THEY FIT INTO THE CLINICAL TRIAL TEAMS?

'There are no problems, only solutions.'

—JOHN LENNON

I like this quote. I practice it. I start educational sessions with it, and over the years, it became representative of me. My career as a paediatric critical care pharmacist started with it. I was talking to an intensive care staff when the unit director interrupted, asking, 'What is the problem'? and I just blurted out, 'There are no problems, only solutions'. That was the beginning of an eight-year journey—one of the most challenging and rewarding in my career. When I started managing clinical trials, my quotes changed according to the CT service needs. I displayed 'If you change nothing, nothing will change' and 'Failing to plan is planning to fail'. They guided me over the five years that followed.

Are CT pharmacists a fit or misfit with the site clinical teams? This question has intrigued me from the day I started working in the area, and my curiosity led me to further explore and share my experience.

On my first day on the job, there were thirty-plus active CTs at different stages. The numbers of enrolled participants ranged from a few to more than hundreds. There were piles of investigational products returned by participants, awaiting accountability performance. The pharmacy folders appeared messy. The delegations' logs revealed frequent staff moves, with an average stay on the job of four to six months over a period of several years. There was no service planner about upcoming participants' visits requiring IP supply, upcoming monitoring visits, or printed copies of post-monitoring visit reports with the open pharmacy items with due completion dates. There were no records of regular billing for pharmacy services or CT agreements available to refer to about the fees. The very long list of uncompleted tasks unmistakably revealed the provision of a basic scope of trial services, mainly IP dispensing and receiving, and other tasks performed when required or upon CRCs' and CRAs' requests.

The reality was that I had inherited a CT service in distress, but with demand and massive potential for rebuilding and growing. Shortly it became apparent that the previous pharmacists may have felt like misfits and left. You might wonder, *How does one become aware of or experience misfit at work?* Well, clinical trials are managed via multidisciplinary teams, yet I felt like an outsider. The perceived misfit was not personal, but somewhat related to the workplace environment and the established practice of PIs obtaining quick okays directly from the pharmacy senior management. The pharmacists before me may have attempted to cure it, but if unsuccessful, the next best option would have been to move to another area or leave for good.

A broader involvement of CT pharmacists in the various CTs aspects can compensate them for missing out on other informative sessions, training, or conferences, such as investigators' meetings offered to PIs and CRCs. Sadly, pharmacists are not usually encouraged to attend those meetings, which is a considerable disadvantage, as it enforces them to create the prescriptions, dispensing summaries, and IP administration instructions for new CTs, only by self-reading provided materials. Frequently, the information in the IP handling manuals is incomplete, necessitating gathering further information. The issues surrounding IP manuals and proposed solutions are itemised in Chapter 9.

Delphine Girard et al., in the article 'How to Improve the Implementation of Academic Clinical Pediatric Trials Involving Drug Therapy? A Qualitative Study of Multiple Stakeholders' reveals that 'pharmacists often described participation in a clinical trial as "working in distress" due to their late involvement in the process. They felt the pharmaceutical issues were often considered of secondary importance'.[9]

So, CT pharmacist's non-inclusion is a problem that requires action, such as establishing presence or credibility and developing more personalised professional relations with the clinical research team members and stakeholders.

Principal investigators are not automatically familiar with pharmacy CT service structure and operational processes. Thus, they may appear insensitive towards possible pharmaceutical issues or perceive them as non-important. Hospital physicians' experience with the pharmacy is often restricted to the common knowledge that pharmacists supply, compound, and dispense medicines to patients and provide advice on their use. For example, many internal and external stakeholders have limited insight into pharmacy trial services and costs; thus, they may not be considered or anticipated. However, in a self-funded pharmacy CT service model, continuous support of under-or non-funded research projects may lead to unsustainable quantity and quality of trial-related services provided by overworked and stressed-out pharmacists who are physically unable to be efficient. High staff turnover is an unavoidable consequence. It is a matter of weighing the pros and cons of supporting underfunded research and keep PIs happy or lose irreplaceable, experienced pharmacists for the wrong reasons and further narrow the scope and capability of the pharmacy CT service.

The COVID-19 crisis once again confirmed that pharmacists had been left out due to the gap of awareness of their specific needs or to the habitual non-inclusion or lack of time to participate in the decision making of adjusting clinical trial practices towards remote and virtual operations.

Next, I will briefly explore the misfit concept and how different people approach and deal with it, as the topic is not restricted to research pharmacists. Anyone can experience it. I share the strategies I used because by successfully resolving it, I stayed longer than anticipated, dedicated more time to building bridges with stakeholders, and enjoyed my work. An essential component in resolving perceived or actual misfit is to focus on the work instead of on the misfit itself.

THE FIT/MISFIT PERCEPTION

Over almost one hundred years, researchers have recognised the fit/misfit as a complex foundation of work-related outcomes. On an individual level, a good fit is associated with team cohesion and job satisfaction. For years, a misfit has been described as 'incompatibility', 'incongruence of person and environment', at 'the lower end of the fit scale'.[10] A large volume of research has established that an employee's usual reactions to low level fit or high level misfit is a poor attitude and high turnover.[11]

Misfit perceptions can be triggered or exacerbated by social signals sent by others or when an individual's professional role is not enhanced in the anticipated way. On the fit-misfit continuum, *fit* is the positive end and *misfit* is the negative end.

The thinking processes of how different people may approach the misfit scenario are as follows:

- Fit/misfit perception
- Assessment of social signals and triggers
- Misfit confirmed
- Plan of action
- *Do I resign and leave?*

After deciding to resign and move on, the strategies either demand an internal transfer or start actively looking for jobs elsewhere. Both are not immediate solutions, as it takes time to find a new job or organise an internal transfer. However, viewing the situation as temporary with a future end date, people tend to distance themselves from work or even take pride in being a misfit to reduce emotional pain and discomfort. Research shows that adopting inauthentic behaviours as a coping mechanism to mitigate misfit-related negative emotions can create even higher levels of stress and exhaustion.[12]

After deciding to stay, corrective strategies are either making changes to the workplace, focussing on personal changes, or both. For example, feeling like a misfit requires correction because it is a problem, motivating people to address it and either act or react to it.

I believe it is a resolvable problem, as I felt like a misfit with some teams, but a good fit with other teams. Thus, I started exploring what changes I could make.

Personal changes start with self-assessment and self-reflection, whether aspects of personal behaviour, feelings, attitudes, or skills contribute to the perceived misfit. Often, self-changes are all that is required. However, in my case, the misfit was caused by workplace flaws; thus, personal changes would have been unreasonable, even undesirable.

The literature informs that often people who cannot resolve or mitigate the misfit tend to disengage from their work, which is demoralising and leads to additional strain caused by both the misfit and the reduced professional engagement. Furthermore, unsuccessful misfit resolutions nearly always lead to increased frustration and higher levels of perceived misfit and cause employees to leave for the wrong reasons.

Although a misfit is generally perceived as a negative state, research confirms my personal experiences to result in positive outcomes. Building workplace relationships leads to personal behaviour changes, growth, development, and new skill acquisitions. Over the years, I had the privilege to work with great PIs.

The most satisfying experiences have been when we all teamed up towards the common goal—a successful trial execution.

In practice, not everyone will successfully resolve the misfit, and that is perfectly all right because changing a work environment is hard; it requires systematic effort, patience, and time. Also, the workplace needs to be either supportive or open to changes. Joyce Brothers' quote, *'If you change nothing, nothing changes'*, has guided me throughout the journey and ascertained what I stand for—*Evolving the Dinosaur.*

LESSONS LEARNED:

- Misfit has long been viewed as a stressor to which people respond using coping and defence mechanisms to reduce the strain it causes.[13]
- Yu, in 2009, suggested some employees get motivated to resolve misfit. They consider it as an opportunity for change and for personal growth; thus, it can have positive consequences.[14]
- Some people respond to social signals of a misfit by adopting inauthentic behaviours as a coping mechanism to mitigate related negative emotions, but that can create even higher levels of stress and exhaustion.
- The negative consequences of an unresolved misfit are feelings of isolation, fatigue, and increased stress.

CLINICAL TRIAL PHARMACISTS AS A PERFECT FIT

When included in all new trial steps from start to end, pharmacists become better versed with the protocol requirements and participant details, therefore able to provide more comprehensive support, resulting in numerous benefits:

- Providing initial funding quotes to PIs and assistance with IP dosing regimens, administration, and addressing possible compliance issues
- Prompt identification of potential issues and finding solutions to avoid future setbacks
- Pre-planning trial necessities ahead of its commencement
- Meeting legal and regulatory compliance requirements
- Prearranging pharmacy matters for better service delivery
- Resolving staffing issues, according to demands
- Timely administrative task completion
- Early assessment and resolution of expectations to avoid future obstacles
- Early communication of anticipated safety risks and their mitigation

If it is not already an established practice in a pharmacy CT service, creating new or adjusting existing research policies and procedures that mandate PIs to provide a quote for the pharmaceutical part of their research projects signed by a CT pharmacist, along with funding applications, should be considered. From experience, it improved CT service planning, led to smoother trials execution and healthier collaborative and professional relations, all positively contributing towards *Evolving the Dinosaur.*

BOTTOM-UP VERSUS TOP-DOWN DECISION MAKING

Which management style is healthier for pharmacy CT services: the top-down or bottom-up approach? Why do CT pharmacists benefit from bottom-up decision making in the research area? Since they are GCP-certified, better versed in the individual trial requirements, the service operational and financial performance, and future needs than pharmacy top management, they should lead and work directly with research teams and external parties towards more efficient delivery of services. In this rapidly growing area of the pharmacy, individual decision-making power matters for prompt solutions.

The top-down chain of command practice, where upper management determines pharmacy CT operations, can negatively impact services delivery, mainly due to inadequate communication and coordination with CT pharmacists. Top management is not required to undertake GCP training, and if not well acquainted with the trials' requirements and agreements, they can provide inappropriate task prioritisation or directions.

For example, they may request a monitoring visit immediately to clear a space currently occupied by a large volume of participants IP returns. However, that is impossible because the CT agreement provides for no less than three monthly monitoring visits. Explaining protocol requirement and trial agreements clauses to justify why we can or cannot do something hinders service efficiency. Pharmacy CT service is a specialised area where the top-down approach frequently fails to develop enough commitment. However, combining top-down and bottom-up approaches allows for better facilitation of change implementation.

LESSONS LEARNED:

- Bottom-up approach allowed early management of unrealistic expectations of delivering timely and safe services on short notice. For example, the new pharmacy CT set-up cannot be completed before all identified challenges are resolved.
- Assessing and confirming pharmacy CT service capacity

and capability before each new trial was crucial for their efficient implementation, as the service is utilised by external sponsors and internal investigators from various medical specialties.
- Accommodating high volume research at any point in time, against limited human resources, primarily when local IP/placebo manufacturing was required, has led to dispensing delays and increased staff distress about compromising participants' continuous supply.

A PROVEN FRAMEWORK FOR CROSS-FUNCTIONAL COLLABORATION AND WORKFLOW STREAMLINING

Collaboration is the new normal in workplaces. Team members no longer expect to work cut off from one another. Effective collaboration improves efficiency and increases productivity through frequent communication about things that matter.

How is cross-functional workflow with integrated IPs dispensing into participants' clinical visits achieved?

When designing workflow, keep in mind that it does not need to be complicated. For example, the starting point to get familiar with a participant visit for a particular trial was to collect information about what would be performed and when the team members would complete it. Once I knew what time the participant arrived, the sequence of tests, scans, etc. and, when their appointment with the PI was, the gathered information guided the workflow design. One additional detail was to pay attention to any undesirable impact on other team members.

The next steps were implementing, evaluating, and adjusting until achieving desired results *with measurable outcomes*. For example, do patients wait for their IPs at the end of a clinical visit? For how long? If reducing wait time is the goal, what can we change and how much can we reduce it—from half an hour to fifteen minutes or none? Wait time reduction and total elimination are achievable and described in Chapter 6.

I have been privileged to collaborate with teams based on sound professional relationships, high trust, reciprocity, and interdependence. However, from not-so-great experiences, I also know that relationships are vulnerable and can easily be disrupted or even destabilised when the withholding of information or resources is introduced.

PHARMACY ORGANISED EXPERIENTIAL VISITS

I had a rough start in the CT area. Speedy changes were required, so I began the rebuilding journey with meet and greet visits with the research teams, which I call 'experiential visits', or learning by experience. The primary purpose of these visits was to bring humanity back into the clinical trials area by exploring how to minimise research team members' and customers' dissatisfaction, to eliminate wait time for pharmacy services, and to implement other possible improvements. Hospital pharmacies cater to external customers and internal health professionals. In the absence of a separate window for each customer's type, a nurse keen to help a patient and reduce their wait time by personally handing in a prescription or collecting dispensed medicines would have to queue like everyone else and wait until her turn comes. That can be fifteen minutes or longer, depending on how busy the pharmacy is. IP prescriptions were handed to the person on the window, then passed on to me without any information about who got them in, how urgent they were, or when they would be collected.

The idea to try experiential visits came about after some brainstorming what would allow me to quickly reach the research team members and make a collective decision about the best course of action to increase efficiency. That is how it started—a hypothesis that an introductory CT pharmacy visit with the trial team members, can increase effectiveness and participants satisfaction by direct communication and collaboration to coordinate various trial tasks. Next was to test it in practice. The initiative was welcomed and appreciated because many of the invitees had not been inside the pharmacy before. That is how the introductory pharmacy tours were conceived and became a standard practice.

Note: the described practice happened pre-COVID-19, but it easily can be adjusted to virtual visits or meetings.

During the visit, the discussions were centred around:

1. Pharmacy CT service operational and management style
2. Lessons learned from the past
3. Current state
4. Re-imagining the future
5. Opportunities to improve new CTs planning and decision making

Similarly, other internal stakeholders either visited the pharmacy or were visited personally to discuss the operational processes, focusing on synchronising processes and streamlining workflows.

In summary, the experiential visits initiative was initially time-consuming, but the future benefits outweighed the time expended.

It was a successful initiative, which was gradually adopted as a standard practice. With clinical trials numbers growing exponentially and corresponding growth of communication ratio of one pharmacist interacting with hundreds of internal and external parties, it was the best option and the most efficient way to build more personalised professional relations with the team members. The approach had the additional benefit for PIs to feel comfortable enough to visit the pharmacy and discuss participants, trials progress or just drop off an IP prescription.

PHARMACISTS' EDUCATIONAL PRESENTATIONS

Additionally, CT pharmacists can run an educational presentation to institutional PIs/SIs and CRCs to deepen their understanding of CT pharmacy services and research pharmacist's functions, practices, and challenges throughout project implementation and propose pragmatic solutions for overcoming them. It is the fastest path to get the message across to many internal parties at once. Even a fifteen–twenty-minute presentation, combined with local ethics and governance educational sessions for internal researchers, proved to be an effective way of raising awareness and gaining collaborative support.

THE 'RECHARGING BREAKS'

'Recharging breaks' are the time spent away from a pharmacy for face to face meetings with research team members regarding participants' visits, workflow adjustments, participants' IP compliance, and other essential matters, or to make a brief appearance in the team meetings to discuss or address pharmaceutical issues.

The recharging breaks positively impacted closing the communication and collaboration gap and helped me achieve my goal—to be part of well-functioning clinical teams and downright included in relevant correspondence and decision making.

THE 2CS FRAMEWORK WITH REDEFINED PROFESSIONAL RELATIONS

Naturally, research pharmacists work in an accommodating, cooperative, and collaborative manner with diverse research stakeholders. Still, the next level was building a high-trust relationship to improve efficiency, productivity, and agility.

Paediatric clinical trials are theoretically an interprofessional teamwork effort. However, to achieve true interprofessional collaboration, clinical site' teams, research pharmacists, trial monitors, and other stakeholders must learn from each other and learn about the work that other members perform. Furthermore, that is the only avenue to put the participants first and make trial implementation safer and more cost-effective.

We, as a team, have different skillsets and expertise areas, but we share the same goal—to complete the clinical trials on hand under the PI's leadership. Thus, a clinical site succeeds or fails as a team.

Even though collaboration, as a concept, is widely overused, surprisingly, there is a vague understanding of how to implement, measure, and improve collaborative working.

My experience in achieving successful collaboration has been in three essential areas: coordination, cooperation, and shared decision making. Firstly, working together towards shared goals, we work in coordination. Secondly, to function well, as an interdisciplinary team, we need to understand other team members roles and appreciate their contributions, meaning we work in cooperation. Thirdly, to practice shared decision-making, we communicate openly, challenge each other without fear of disregard, and respect the interprofessional power balance.

Usually, interprofessional relationships in which all members work equitably together are cultivated over time. So, the next logical question is, how we can develop humble interprofessional relationships in clinical trials promptly? Of course, we all perform different activities, but we benefit from each other's input at every stage by coordinating them.

The practical benefit of coordination was an efficient, effective, and better way to manage the trial risks, such as, but not limited to, IP storage, dispensing, administration, blinding and unblinding, treatment allocation, and any other risks to participants, staff, and the organisation.

What were the benefits of collaboration?

Presently, collaboration remains the 'go to' strategy for generating collective impact. Some of the benefits are self-evident. For example, we leverage the synergies of working together and complete complex clinical trials more efficiently and cost-effectively.

Theory and practice are aligned in that qualitatively collaboration leads to improved health outcomes, quality care, sharing knowledge and information on best practices and enhanced decision-making. Quantitatively, as outlined in the measurement plan further in the book, collaborative teamwork led to reduced length of clinical visits, cost-saving and improved compliance with the protocol, regulatory standards, quality audit results, and improved trial data management.

Trial participants' safety, engagement, experience, and satisfaction are highly dependent on collaborative culture and teamwork. Additionally, it is well recognised that organisations fostering a collaborative culture enjoy high staff retention and fulfilment.

Other benefits include greater perceptions of inclusion, empowerment, and recognition because collaborative teams' structure is generally more horizontal rather than hierarchical.

Another intriguing question is whether we can measure collaboration. My exploration of the costs and benefits of cooperation affirmed that it is challenging to identify and quantify it. Research suggests that estimating the total costs of collaboration, including the lost opportunity costs, and determining if a future collaboration is the best possible option, is hard to measure. While team behaviour can be measured with questionnaires to obtain individual perceptions about collaborative behaviour, its direct measuring appears to be challenging to quantify accurately and time-consuming because behaviours required direct observational studies.

My subsequent exploration focused on how we can collaborate more efficiently, effectively, and achieve desired results, but in a more relaxing mode. Theoretically, a motivated and successful team has members who trust each other, are accountable to one another, accept their interdependency and differences, and feel safe to behave in open and transparent ways.

In clinical research, interprofessional teamwork between external and internal stakeholders is complex due to the differing priorities and responsibilities. Thus, a new framework with redefined professional relations is required more than ever. Coordination and cooperation are the basic foundation of targeted collaboration to improve efficiency and increase productivity. Sharing ideas, insights, and trial matters or concerns as equal team members was an efficient way to close the gap between clinical site team members and other interprofessional trial stakeholders to build a more vital, awareness-based collaboration.

Open team discussions and evaluations of research projects changing priorities led to avoiding impediments. Clinical sites teams incorporate a diversity of knowledge, skills, and training to work together with research participants and their family, towards delivering superior services.

It was also essential to keep in mind that to collaborate effectively, we have to work on our collaborative skill. As developing another skill, it takes time and effort to learn about the needs, expectations, and capabilities of collaboration, find areas of agreement, reach an agreement on what and how to work together, and finally, establish appropriate communication processes.

Naturally, we expect cost savings from collaboration because we work in more connected or integrated ways. Still, research by Keast et al. shows cost benefits failure between 50-70 per cent due to process failures, such as not reaching the necessary strength of relationship, collaboration taking place in the wrong forum, and insufficient collaborative competency or commitment to work in new or different ways.[15]

Collaboration demands strong relationships based on high

trust, reciprocity, and interdependence. Research shows that it takes time to build and nurture a relationship- between three to five years. Collaborative relationships are vulnerable and can easily be disrupted by not sharing information or resources. Collaborators may have conflicting priorities or may even resent being tasked with the extra work required of collaboration. Collaborative initiatives involve spending time on them, which is a personal cost, often using personal time, resources, and networks to get collaborative endeavours underway and keep them going. What do all these facts mean? It means that paediatric drug development, research stakeholders, hospitals and healthcare services conducting clinical trials should consider setting up systems and resources to support collaboration, such as workshops, training, and better systems for data and information sharing.

EDUCATION AND SKILLS TO MANAGE PHARMACY CLINICAL TRIALS SERVICE: THE MISSING INGREDIENT

Currently, there are no internal or external basic or advanced courses teaching paediatric research methodology and logistics. Paediatric clinical pharmacist residency programs exist and are becoming quite popular, but similar ones for paediatric research are less common, and it is not a core subject in the pharmacy curriculum. A few programs offer a specialised research career track to pharmacy students after completing a PharmD via postgraduate fellowships.

The lack of educational programs teaching research principles and practice skills limits the entry point for new graduates into this specialised area. Official, standardised certification or demonstration and simulation-based paediatric research educational programs would be beneficial, and indeed, we will see more of them in the future, but until it happens, experienced paediatric clinical trials pharmacists should continue acting as the primary source of knowledge dissemination, mentoring, onboarding, and training other pharmacy staff.

Girard D. and colleagues in 2013 pointed out the 'need for the development of research paediatric pharmacists, trained in providing an early pharmaceutical expertise, including making recommendations consistent with the methodological constraints'. The authors suggest that 'most of the pharmaceutical problems could be prevented by performing pharmaceutical feasibility assessments during the development of the study protocol. The pharmaceutical aspects are intrinsically tied to trial methodology and implementation and must therefore be examined particularly by involving research pharmacists at early stages of study conception'.[16]

Before commencing work in the clinical trials area, pharmacists must complete GCP training, consisting of thirty- to forty-five-minute modules, taking around three to six hours to complete. That is insufficient for new researchers to gain a complete grasp and understanding of these international quality standards and regulations for clinical trials in human subjects. Minimal knowledge cannot possibly translate into practical confidence.

Would it be more beneficial for new pharmacists, trial coordinators, and other researchers to do at least one comprehensive GCP training, preferably at the beginning of their career? Yes, because each stakeholder must have a complete understanding of their roles and obligations and how their part relates to or may affect others.

TRAINING THE TRAINER

CT pharmacists are trained on individual trials via face to face, online courses, and more frequently by reading/self-training before training other pharmacy staff, as required. They must first manage their own training and then disseminate the information to others. Training must be documented on original pharmacy training logs and filed in a pharmacy folder.

Templates of a pharmacy CT training log and delegation logs can be obtained from my website: www.paediatricpharma.com or via email at violetford@paediatricpharma.com. They can be modified, individualised, and adjusted to suit specific training areas.

THE SKILLS

'Excellence is not a skill, it's an attitude'.

—RALPH MARSTON

Currently, the demand for paediatric-experienced clinical trials/research pharmacists exceeds the supply. Experienced and advanced paediatric clinical practitioners are less likely to seek employment in this specific area because of the limited career progression.

There are no published, standardised requirements about specific skills or additional qualifications for providing clinical trial services. General practice standards suggest GCP and Good Manufacturing Practice (GMP) training as the only essential certifications. A fundamental level of knowledge of research methodology or postgraduate qualification is desirable but not a prerequisite.

There is a lack of courses, programs or publications teaching paediatric pharmacy CT service assessment and management, change management, tracking effectiveness, or service scaling and increasing its performance and efficiency. While IP handling and other trial-related tasks are a pharmacist's responsibilities, an absence of effective CT service management may negatively affect delivering prompt services to hundreds of trials and their participants, managed at the site level simultaneously. I wish I had some directions or guidance when I started, from someone who had made the journey of managing an understaffed CT service with an exponentially increasing work volume.

So, what skills are necessary for a pharmacy managed CT service which manages the individual trials?

COMMUNICATION SKILLS

While communication skills are a generic requirement, CT/research work's nature requires a swift change from scientific language to plain and back. We communicate with many different internal and external parties, such as PIs, CRCs; CRAs; sponsors; pharmaceutical company representatives; auditors, regulatory, governance and ethics officers, trial participants, parents/caregivers, and other parties involved in research. Those people come from different backgrounds, with various levels of education and understanding of research principles or the pharmacist's role and services. As a result, we may frequently need to change from technical language to ordinary instantaneously and back, depending on the audience—for example, providing information to a PI, a participant, and their parent in one room. The language to the PI is professional; to the parent, non-technical; and to the child, maybe playful, depending on their age and understanding.

MULTITASKING AND MANAGING DEADLINES

Clinical trials require developing and employing *multitasking and managing deadlines* due to the nature of the work. In addition, interprofessional tasks and duties' dependence are inherent in clinical research, as different parties perform different tasks. For example, a delay in preparing a pharmacy budget may affect the site trial commencement.

Years of experience in the area, combined with *volume and variety of trials managed*, broaden our understanding of the comprehensive research picture, which is different from the routine pharmacy practice. Furthermore, to increase service effectiveness, implement change management, practice improvements, and culture change, *personal virtues* are fundamental for establishing our credibility and trust with other hospital staff, research team members, patients, sponsors, and people from other research organisations.

HIGH LEVEL CUSTOMER SERVICE

There is an expectation of a *high level of customer service,* which is not hard to achieve with the right attitude. Generally, experience is desirable but usually not essential if the *right mindset and an aptitude to learn* are in place. Often those qualities are more than sufficient to succeed.

SELF-LEARNING AND READING

'Formal education will make you a living; self-education will make you a fortune'.

—JIM ROHN

An aptitude for learning is sufficient to succeed in the clinical trials area, as a *great deal of the learning is self-learning and reading.* An example is to review, assess, and comment on a new protocol scientifically.

We learn how to learn what we need to know that pharmacy school did not teach at some point in our professional lives. I am not aware of a more effective method than self-directed learning by diagnosing our learning needs, designing, and assessing our learning experiences. It requires a planned and structured approach, dedication, and most importantly, self-motivation to do so due to the limited free time at work. It can be discouraging, if it is not a work requirement or is unrelated to the job description and does not lead to an instant promotion or appreciation by teammates or management. I never anticipated that as a pharmacist, I would need to master other disciplines, such as business management and leadership, negotiation, process mapping, change management, workflow streamlining, efficiencies and effectiveness, and culture change, to name a few.

Are there any benefits of spending personal time on self-learning? Yes. It has positively impacted my credibility with on-the-spot problem-solving gaining the respect of being efficient, well-versed, and knowledgeable—a subject matter expert.

By investing time to expand our knowledge bank, we become valuable team contributors, fulfil our responsibilities, and support others to do so.

PLANNING AND TAKING PREVENTATIVE MEASURES

Good planning and taking preventative measures are valuable skills.

'If you fail to plan, you are planning to fail'.

—BENJAMIN FRANKLIN

Pharmacy CT Service planning encompasses delivering the daily core services from their current state and developing an action plan to an improved future state. It encompasses baseline assessment, problem identification and prioritisation, action plan, and measuring and tracking the outcomes. Lack of planning affects the delivery of prompt and high quality services. Without preventative measures, a lot of effort is directed only towards putting out fires. Failing to identify or attend to and treat problems straight away is not an intelligent decision, and neither is problem avoidance. Unresolved issues quickly become more challenging to contain and consume extra time and effort.

Applied skills, perspective view, and proactive actions with continuous assessment of what does and does not work are vital to collecting and analysing relevant data points and measuring the success of executed changes and improvements.

SYSTEMS, PROCEDURES, AND DOMAIN KNOWLEDGE

Systems, procedures, and domain knowledge are prerequisites for developing CT service policies and standard operational procedures (SOPs), which are provided to sponsors and CROs as required. Well designed and correctly describing the actual practice, SOPs are directly reflective of the CT service credibility.

STRONG ACTIVE LISTENING

Active listening is a crucial skill for personal and professional success. Research confirms that pharmacy services are strongly influenced by customers' perceptions of how well pharmacists listened to them.

FLEXIBILITY

Being flexible to consistently accommodate unexpected trial-related tasks and fit them in with other team members' duties adds value to participants' convenience and CT service. Humble communication encourages team members to weave their clinical duties with pharmacy dispensing to streamline workflows.

The immediate benefit of achieving an on-the-spot fit resolution is rewarding. The long-term benefits of being flexible are increased team cohesion, trust, and gaining their commitment. Flexibility drives people to find solutions that work for everyone else involved.

Pharmacy trial tasks are customised to meet protocol requirements; thus, exceptional *organisational skills and attention to detail* are necessary.

Desirable skills for successful management of paediatric clinical trial service fall under three categories:

- What we know or *knowledge skills* is our domain knowledge.
- What we can do or *applied skills*, including problem-solving, evidence gathering, evaluation, analysis, planning, workflow management, feedback and training, communication, advice, influence, engagement, and collaboration.
- *Behaviour skills* define how we act and how that applies to our professional and ethical conduct.

CONTINUING EDUCATION AND PROFESSIONAL GROWTH

CT pharmacists handle excessive administrative and clerical work, such as manual recording or electronic entries in multiples logs/Interactive Response Technology (IRT), scanning/faxing, or emailing various paperwork to multiple external parties. This work is in addition to service management and the standard IP management and handling. Workplaces encourage professional development, but for CT/research pharmacists, continuing education supporting their professional growth is distinct and aligned with their job.

Further education may include but is not restricted to:

- Gaining or expanding expertise on paediatric disease states related to current and forthcoming CTs.
- Accumulating in-depth knowledge on the current best treatments compared to the investigational products.
- Developing educational materials for site personnel on proper handling and use of new investigational products.
- Gaining or expanding knowledge on pharmacy operations, institutional policies, procedures, and guidelines.
- Scientific literature research on specific topics, including IP doses, administration instructions, and side effects, as required.

CT/research pharmacists have distinctive positioning and multidimensional contributions throughout trial implementation; thus, it is essential for them to continually update or expand their knowledge on the latest advances in pharmacological science.

STAFFING REQUIREMENTS FOR *EVOLVING THE DINOSAUR*

Currently, the supply of pharmacists exceeds the number of available jobs in hospital pharmacies, thus, the sense that there are not too many opportunities available. Employment trends are based on variable factors, such as geographic region, hospital pharmacy setting, experience, skillset, and demand.

Following the incentives and initiatives for boosting paediatric research, demand for pharmacy CT services has grown and continues to rise exponentially. However, even if the revenue generated by a pharmacy CT service can self-fund additional pharmacist positions, hospital administrators' lack of immediate response to employ additional staff prevents CT services from expanding naturally. Delayed response to a sudden increase in demand of services or understaffing caused by employees' turnover affects the seamless management of trial pharmaceuticals and the delivery of quality services.

Often, the gap between the number of pharmacists employed and the number required for safe trial related tasks management can be vast and over extended periods. Although self-funding inability should not be considered a justifiable reason for understaffing because there are other cost savings by treating hospital patients with investigational products. For example, differed costs for not treating those patients while participating in clinical trials and costs avoidance from not purchasing study drugs. While the topic of institutional cost savings and reducing drug expenditure by treating patients within clinical trials is essential for hospital administrators, an economic evaluation of pharmacy CT services is not within the scope of this book.

Chronic understaffing can be a problem in any workplace, but it can have weighty consequences in healthcare. Staffing issues can be grouped around four points:

1. *Delayed response* to increased service demands, leading to dangerous levels of understaffing. Approval processes and justification requirements about the necessity of new job positions are way too bureaucratic and lengthy.
2. *Shortage of experienced paediatric pharmacists.* It has been noted that with new job position openings, there are limited applications by experienced paediatric pharmacists and an oversupply of new graduates who lack experience in both paediatrics and research.
3. *Limited understanding of the nature of clinical trials and research work* by pharmacy management and hospital administrators. Lack of support results in higher rates of staff turnover and diminished retaining of expertise.
4. *Absence of established staff-determining metrics* and lack of regulatory standards about the accepted volume of clinical trial tasks per one full-time pharmacist applied nationally or internationally. Currently, it remains unsolved.

Hospital administrators can be hesitant to fund additional full-time pharmacists to CT services because they fear increased costs without a return on investment, but the contributions of CT/research pharmacists can and should be assessed and justified by other more appropriate metrics than cost alone.

OVERWORKED AND HIGHLY STRESSED

Research shows that pharmacists, with time, eventually emerge as overworked and highly stressed due to insufficient staffing levels. They often work in isolation, without breaks or necessary resources, and feel invisible to the outside world, leading to shortcuts in processes and subsequent increases in protocol deviations or medication errors.

There are no established *paediatric clinical trial staffing standards* or regulations about an employee's threshold per service-related metrics.

There are suggestions that staffing structure and levels required for managing adult clinical trials services should be determined by four major factors:

1. Number of active CTs
2. Complexity and phase of the CTs
3. Rate at which new CTs are being opened and closed
4. Number of recruited participants

While those four factors appear reasonable, there is no acumen about the determination process, the frequency of metrics collection, assessments, and analyses of collected data, or implementation responsibility of data- confirmed staffing requirements, especially for CT services, where understaffing is a norm rather than an exception.

Can specialised paediatric hospitals delivering CT services establish workload methods or formulas to determine appropriated staffing levels based on employees' workload tolerance tests? Maybe! However, presently, this rapidly expanding pharmacy area is not yet subject to standardised staffing, nationally or internationally, nor it is based on specific, validated metrics or regulatory standards upon accepted levels of staffing. Until a solution is found, the number of CT pharmacists in some hospitals will probably remain unrelated to the number of active CTs, their complexity, the number of enrolled participants per trial, the number of budgets negotiated, the number of invoices raised, and service revenue, or investigational product errors prevented, the list could go on and on.

WHAT DOES THIS MEAN FOR CLINICAL TRIAL PHARMACISTS?

It means that the workload could get significantly higher than the physical ability that an employee can handle. Published research shows that in a Korean adult hospital, the workload was up to 2.3 times higher for the number of pharmacists involved.[17]

It appears that staffing challenges are under-recognised and yet to be identified and considered. In addition, the lack of pharmacy administrative staff to handle clerical duties, while pharmacists focus on managing the service, is not accounted for either. A busy service is prone to an unhealthy communication ratio of one pharmacist to hundreds of research personnel irrespective of being in person or via phone/email. Often, pharmacists do not have uninterrupted time. Managing a massive number of participant visits with various requirements concurrently with countless interruptions, distractions, and multitasking is concerning due to children's unique safety risks, coupled with limited safety and efficacy information about IPs. The Institute for Safe Medication Practices recently reported that each interruption is associated with a 12.7 per cent increase in medication errors for nurses. Similarly, CT pharmacists would benefit from a 'safe zone' to work, with minimum distractions or interruptions to avoid dispensing errors and compromising participant safety and data integrity.[18]

Paediatric clinical trial services tend to accommodate a large volume of internal and external research projects, while the actual number of employees remains unchanged. The imbalance between demand and the ability to support the demand requires new, creative ways of increasing personal and service efficiencies. Otherwise, the CT service will default to the provision of basic trial management. However, what happens when an understaffed CT service dramatically expands? Can CT pharmacists continue to provide value-added services and quality care?

A literature search on paediatric CT/research pharmacists' impact on participant outcomes or evidence of any other measurable effect did not identify published articles or investigations related to the topic. Unlike the well-established positive role clinical pharmacists play in healthcare cost-saving and enhancing patient outcomes, no publications show a similar measurable impact of CT pharmacists on research participants. The lack of data could be related to time and resources limitations that prevent pharmacists from performing relevant research projects, measuring outcomes, and publishing the results. Future research and publications are required to establish measurable effects of the pharmacist services provided to patients enrolled in clinical trials.

A few articles on adult CT services identified lack of time, support, and training as critical barriers to participation in research.

I determined that pharmacists' moderate interest in CT/research stems from a limited professional direction in career advancement. Pharmacists with prior experience in the area, or those appreciating the benefits of research discoveries towards future patient care improvements, are more primed to join the research community than those who do not have previous experience or understanding. The shared belief that clinical research is part of a pharmacist's professional responsibilities and that new treatments are essential for improving patient care may not be sufficient to attract young pharmacists.

Knowledge expansion and professional growth in this area are restricted. Understaffing, lack of time, and funding constraints are the main reasons for CT pharmacists' inability to attend in-person or virtual paediatric CT conferences, symposiums, and other educational events. One may argue that the protocols outline the relevant tasks, but the information provided by sponsors/CROs is enough for a basic CT administration. To effectively manage a large unit, a senior or advanced practitioner is required to assess new trial protocols scientifically and to detect any variances between IP administration instructions in protocols and best paediatric practices or identify safety issues or other inconsistencies.

HOW MANY HATS DOES A MANAGING PHARMACIST WEAR?

Pharmacists managing CT services do not operate in a consistent and predictable work environment. The job scope is broad and often necessitates employing multidimensional skills, assuming responsibilities outside the job description parameters, changing many hats to attain value-added services and transformational changes of healthcare delivery targeted at *Evolving the Dinosaur*.

For successful service management, effective time and conflict management skills, the ability to understand various healthcare professionals' perspectives, and lead interprofessional research teams are necessary.

The key responsibilities of a service managing pharmacist may include:

- CT service leadership and management
- Operational duties
- CT / investigational product responsibilities
- Educational responsibilities
- Performance appraisals of other research team members and support staff
- Financial and revenue-generating opportunities
- Administrative responsibility
- Medication and participant safety
- Risk mitigation
- Supervisory duties
- Facilitating rapport with other paediatric CT services, PIs, CRCs, other research officers, sponsors, and CROs
- IP and trial information provision
- Intra and interprofessional collaboration

The list is not comprehensive but is reasonably revealing of what it takes to manage a CT service successfully and why its staffing needs should be based on a well-developed operational plan, capturing each service's actual duties and responsibilities individually.

Undoubtedly, *one size does not fit all.*

CHAPTER THREE

Chaotic Paediatric Clinical Trials Service

'It's not understaffing—it's bonus work'.

—DR. EVIL

Paediatric pharmacist-managed CT services are fast-expanding areas but not yet subject to standardised or validated metrics for determining staffing needs. Some of the main reasons a service can become chaotic for intermittent periods of time are as follows:

- Steady or sudden increase in demand for services. For example, vast but unsupported service expansion leads to an imbalance between commitments and available resources.
- Lack of appropriate level of dedicated pharmacy staff to the area or available to step in when required.
- Lack of accurate, data-driven CT service planning.
- Lack of validated metrics for service capacity assessment before committing to facilitate new CTs.
- Limited support of the CT/research service by pharmacy management.

- Lack of strong leadership or in-depth understanding of CT service operational complexities and what it takes to run an organised and efficient service

WHAT DOES CHAOTIC SERVICE LOOK LIKE?

Simply described, a chaotic CT service is an understaffed service, burdened by work overload; employees wrestle with competing deadlines and managing changing priorities while attending to urgent tasks, correspondence, phone queries, incoming dispensing, and shipments. Furthermore, this mix of trial-related tasks and human interactions sprinkled with disruptions and interruptions is managed concurrently. (If only there were a 'drama log' to capture some actual data…)

Chronic understaffing leads to pharmacist burnout and turnover. Those who stay have learned how to maintain control of challenging situations and think of new ways to tackle problems. Reasonable tactics, such as operational process modifications, change management, increasing efficiencies, and leveraging paediatric clinical best practices are only a *few* examples of what is needed to create a *safe* clinical trials practice.

SOLUTIONS FOR KEEPING CONTROL OF CHAOS

We all want to learn how to keep control of our emotions and thoughts, especially when the situation demands it. Maybe some chaos is good for us. It keeps us alert and improves our abilities. However, this topic is not light reading, so let me humour you for a minute with my three rules of handling chaos. I do not claim that they are innovative (some readers may have already used them), but they are practical:

- Rule number one: Do not freak out.
- Rule number two: Do not resign yet.
- Rule number three: Go ahead and do the work of three.

Keeping in mind that short-term solutions for a service in distress are like band-aids, I had to find long-term solutions that would keep it thriving even in chaos.

It may be easier to design and set up a new pharmacy CT/research service from scratch, but more likely, we find ourselves in an established one, requiring various degrees of transformation. After a quick handover, we try to figure out how things work, and if we are lucky, the service is in a healthy state and does not need much reshaping or reviving.

However, what do we do when that is *not* the case? We commence rebuilding the pharmacy CT/research as a service. Simultaneously, we engage in more efficient and effective work methods, develop new collaboration styles with research team members, and redesign the workflows—all feasible solutions.

While I cannot guarantee success for everyone everywhere, the framework and solutions outlined further in the book led to multiple benefits. I hope to show, rather than tell, what positively impacted the operational and financial performance and efficiency and how I got there. The strategies presented are not in order of importance and can be used individually or concurrently, depending on the service state and needs.

The very first step was to identify problems and opportunities for improvement, supporting my objectives. My goal was to turn around the pharmacy CT service from the periphery *to the forefront* of the hospital research ecosystem and deliver efficient trial management, value-added services, and participant-centred care.

The CT service, as it stood, had bitten off much more than it could chew, along with unsupported expansion, a history of frequent staff turnover, and a lack of experienced staff.

The starting point was managing and overcoming my dissatisfaction and frustration before rebuilding the clinical trials/research as a service. I needed to identify metrics and collect robust data to guide the changes towards a well-organised service with streamlined workflows across all active research projects.

Part 2 of the book is exclusively dedicated to service assessment, metrics, and measurements. However, in the following pages, I share how the communication and collaboration management plan came to life and were implemented. One key priority was establishing cooperative and coordinated interprofessional working relations with other internal and external research stakeholders to nurture the service. The communication and collaboration plan included face to face meetings and cross-functional workflows streamlining.

THE MANAGEMENT PLAN

As previously described, during the first weeks of taking over the service management, the implementation of experiential visits to the CT area with the hospital research community members was set in motion. During those meetings, the service overcommitment, staffing issues, and rescue management plan were discussed. The management plan asserted that new CTs would not gain pharmacy support without the trial pharmacist's participation in the pre-and feasibility assessment for preliminary assessment and ratification. All research projects, including those forthcoming, were entered into a newly created service planning database. The management plan also required that all new trial protocols, investigator's brochures (IBs), and pharmacy manuals were forwarded to the CT pharmacists for review and assessment before any scheduled site's feasibility visit.

The management plan, over time, turned into a success. An increasing number of researchers became familiar with how the pharmacy CT service operates and what was to be communicated and when. The wheels of change management were in motion, moving the service towards the transition phase and into an improved state.

As per the Pareto principle*, 20 per cent of the time spent on communication—emails, phone calls, and face to face or virtual meetings with key stakeholders—accounted for 80 per cent of the improvement in cross-functional team interactions and coordination of CTs activities. It worked for me, and I am optimistic that it can work for others, too, if not already in use.

*The Pareto principle is also known as the 80:20 ratio of cause to effect, meaning the relationship between inputs and outputs is not balanced; 80 per cent of the results come from 20 per cent of the activities.

Establishing professional relations with pharmaceutical companies and sponsors or their representatives is fundamental for pharmacy CT services. Those are better managed individually, depending on the frequency of monitoring visits and trial implementation stage: beginning, mid-trial, or nearly completed. Even though face to face meetings are preferable, courtesy phone calls worked as well. The discussion agenda for external parties is different, but achieving efficiency is impossible without establishing rapport and good working relations. Once an external party is aware of our priorities and how we can help them, all pieces come together towards more productive, well-organised, and more effective trial management.

CRA's priorities are easily accommodated. If pharmacy trial-related tasks are performed and documented accurately, and there are no missing shipping documents, they are satisfied because their visits are shortened. They are grateful for the saved time, much needed for the site trial activities review.

THE ACTION PLAN FOR STREAMLINING WORKFLOWS

The management plan also included *an action plan for streamlining cross-functional team workflows.* Cross-functional team workflow during a participant visit is the way work gets done, as detailed in the protocol. All tests and procedures are performed in sequence. If CT pharmacists know the order of procedures and approximate time, the workflow can be mapped, and IP dispensing can fit in with the visit cycle instead of at the end. Knowing which team members and stakeholders to consult enabled an immediate course of action. Upfront alignment on visit details and how we can work together ensured success. Examining the workflow performance helps identify problems and bottlenecks requiring correction, while measuring its performance guides proper actions, if necessary. I will stop here for now, as what metrics can be used and measured are discussed in Part 2 of the book.

THE MEDICATION SAFETY MITIGATION PLAN

Another essential duty was to establish a *medication safety mitigation plan*. Investigational product safety concerns in paediatric CTs are greater than with registered medicines. The reasons for increased safety risks, including the causes and types, and proposed feasible solutions, are explored in Chapter 4. The topic is important because site CT pharmacists carry out local risk assessments of new IPs and prepare management procedures to minimise identified risks to trial participants, staff, and the institution.

CHAPTER FOUR

Medication Safety in Paediatric Clinical Trials

THE IMPORTANCE

In 2007, the Institute for Safe Medication Practices (ISMP) in Canada defined *medication safety* as the 'freedom from preventable harm with medication use'.

Medication safety received enormous attention during the past few decades because it plays a significant role in patient health and can impact health outcomes and costs to the healthcare system.

Medication safety is not a theoretical concept for paediatric pharmacists because they play an active role in reducing error incidents and improve patient safety and quality use of medicines through established strategies and best practices. Professionally, CT pharmacists are best versed with medication safety principles and routinely carry out local risk assessments of new IPs and prepare risk management procedures to minimise identified risks to trial participants/parents/caregivers, staff, and the institution. Potential sources of risk include, but are not limited to, storage, prescribing, dispensing, aseptic manufacturing, administration, blinding and unblinding and treatment allocation, documentation, cost, and post-trial access to medicines.

Drug development stakeholders are predominantly focused on the new drug safety profiles and clinical efficacy; thus, some specific safety issues may be of a lower priority. Even though clinical sites report actual IP errors and potential risks to local ethics committees and institutional review boards (EC/IRBs), and sponsors, the feedback loop has not yet been closed or resulted in substantial corrective measures.

In contrast to the well-recognised requirements to improve multiple areas of trial protocols to increase safety, IP handling manuals and accountability logs' need for amendments have not been formally addressed. The information inconsistencies or errors in them are neither aligned with paediatric best practices nor promote medication safety. EC/IRBs do not review IP handling manuals or data collection tools, and the feedback process to sponsors is not consistent or standardised.

The current status of pharmacy information resources and accountability logs—both created and provided to site pharmacists by sponsors and CROs, along with some practical remedial solutions—are detailed further in the book under 'Pharmacy Clinical Trial Folder' in Chapter 9.

REASONS FOR MEDICATION ERRORS

Medication errors can occur at any point during the chain of patients' pharmaceutical care—prescribing, transcribing, dispensing, administration, and across healthcare settings. Over the years, pharmacists have formulated various methods and adopted preventative strategies and best practices to reduce them by identifying root causes.

Paediatric patients are at greater risk of medication errors and adverse drug reactions compared to adults.

The main reasons are:

- Paediatric prescribing requires weight-based dose calculations. A miscalculation or incorrect body weight can lead to a dosing error.
- Most registered medicines are available in unit-dose packaging for adults. To prepare and accurately measure doses for children, the original medication dosages need to be altered.
- The need for decimal points leads to common errors known as 'factor of ten errors' or decimal place errors.
- Infants and children are physiologically less able to tolerate medication errors or adverse reactions due to underdeveloped renal and hepatic functions.
- Young children cannot communicate or effectively describe what they are experiencing.
- There are limited references about maximum recommended daily doses in children. The current dose calculation practice is milligrams or micrograms multiplied by body weight (BW), and it should not exceed the maximum adult dose. Note: there are exceptions.
- Lack of paediatric care-trained staff.

TYPES OF MEDICATION ERRORS AND CAUSES

From 2006 through 2007, the MEDMARX database from the

US Pharmacopeia in Rockville, Maryland, shows nearly 2.5 per cent of paediatric medication errors led to patient harm.

The most common types of harmful paediatric medication errors were:

- Improper dose/quantity (37.5 per cent)
- Omission error (19.9 per cent)
- Unauthorised/Incorrect drug (13.7 per cent)
- Prescribing error (9.4 per cent), followed by incorrect administration technique, time, or route of administration, dosage form, or formulation

Medication errors involving paediatric patients were most often caused by:

- Performance deficit (43 per cent)
- Knowledge deficit (29.9 per cent)
- Procedure/protocol not followed (20.7 per cent)
- Miscommunication (16.8 per cent) followed by calculation error, computer entry error, inadequate or lack of monitoring, improper use of pumps, and documentation errors.

Takata et al. concluded that 22 per cent of adverse drug events were preventable, 17.8 per cent could have been identified earlier, and 16.8 per cent could have been mitigated more effectively.[19] I use the percentages of errors by types and causes, as per MEDMARX database throughout the book when addressing medication safety issues and practical solutions.

MEDICATION SAFETY RISKS IN PAEDIATRIC CLINICAL TRIALS

An *investigational product* is a pharmaceutical form of an active ingredient or placebo being tested for safety and effectiveness or used as a reference in a clinical trial. IPs have been tested in a laboratory and approved for testing in humans; thus, *the full knowledge of their toxicity and interactions with other medicine and food may not yet be entirely defined or known.*

Protocol complexity, study design, methodology, and age-specific dosing regimens further increase the safety risks. Furthermore, there is limited regulatory oversight to govern and guide medication safety and error prevention, including a lack of standardised safety practices outlined in the paediatric CT protocols.

What possible risks can be encountered?

INVESTIGATIONAL PRODUCT RISKS

LOOK ALIKE IPS

To maintain trial blinding, visual differentiation between investigational products and placebos should theoretically not exist. The package appearance and font should be the same in colour, shape, and size. However, this leads to look alike products. While it is essential for blinded CTs when participants are provided with multiple strengths to make up a dose, mix-ups happen and usually are discovered too late. IP dose entries on diaries appear correct, but accountability of returned products does not add up. Likewise, in open label trials, where blinding is no longer necessary, the look alike appearance of different IP strengths is not eliminated. Similarly, in dose titration CTs, different strengths are often supplied in look alike containers, which poses the risk of participants being given an incorrect dose. Moreover, it creates storage difficulties. Generally, different strengths of the same IP need to be physically separated.

To prevent dosing errors and for easy differentiation, and to avoid products mix=up at home, CT pharmacists are forced to think of creative ways to keep participants safe while maintaining blinding. Whether manually highlighting the IP strength in a different colour or packaging in separate Ziplock bags, it is an ineffective way to tackle medication safety issues.

Although it is exciting that pharma companies embrace patient centricity, it is also hoped that the integration and initiatives are extended into paediatric drug development. My first-hand experience with looking through participants or their parents/caregivers' eyes is that more frequently than not, they are concerned, apprehensive, or fearful about product mix-ups, administration mistakes, or measuring the doses accurately and even more when they do.

The lesson learned is that CT pharmacists alone cannot solve medication errors related to parents' confusion at home over instructions, IP packaging, expiry dates, measuring tools, and other factors. It requires team effort, involving multiple stakeholders, gaining deep insight into the issues, and *making improvements for safer IP management at home because trial participants' experience does not end when they walk out of the clinical site* with the IP supply or after it is delivered to their homes.

INVESTIGATIONAL PRODUCT NAME SIMILARITIES

Another safety risk is IP name similarity, mainly when multiple trials by the same sponsor are conducted simultaneously at clinical sites. In early phase trials, IP names are created using a number preceded by an abbreviation of the sponsoring company's name. In the absence of a generic or brand name, the IP's name is a string of letters and numbers representing five components: industry code, class, subclass, process indicator code, and the product group. Clinical sites participating in multiple trials by the same sponsor struggle to distinguish the different trials' IPs and to store them appropriately, as IPs with similar names or appearance require physical separation and caution signs/alerts to avoid errors or product mix-ups. Essentially, the sponsor's abbreviated name, industry code, class, and so forth remain the same; therefore, the only difference is the last digits of the identification numbers.

Name similarities can give rise to errors during prescribing, dispensing, and administration. Name inconsistencies have been observed when IPs are assigned generic names. Frequently, while shipping documents and packing slips refer to a product by its new generic name, the physical stock labels continue to reflect the original product code name.

INVESTIGATIONAL PRODUCT LABELS AND PACKAGING

IPs manufactured and shipped to sites by third-party suppliers pose a distinctive set of challenges and risks of errors. Often, either the individual product containers are not labelled, or the opposite, the outer boxes are unlabeled, but the individual containers are. Such practice is unsafe because it is contingent on the on-site CT pharmacists to match products with outer boxes or individual containers labels with packing slips. In paediatric CTs, every possible measure should be taken to reduce or eliminate risks for product mix-ups or errors that may cause harm or affect the data accuracy.

Inadequate or overload of information on IP container labels can increase the risk of errors or restrict the ability to locate essential information when required promptly. Booklet labels on containers are convenient for multinational trials, as the information can be written in up to ten languages and work in different countries simultaneously. While they are intended to increase efficiency and cut costs from a supplier's perspective, site team members find them unsafe and impractical. They are hard to read due to tiny font, not standardised, and challenging to navigate through the language pages to interpret pictograms. Peel off labels are challenging to unpeel and find the required information due to the inherent non-standardised format. Additionally, they are inappropriate for vials, requiring sterile manipulation. Also, children tend to unpeel and rip them off, resulting in accountability and recording compliance difficulties.

Confusing labels with various numbers on them in an unstandardised manner (IP code name, protocol number, lot or batch number, and kit number) impose difficulty determining the meaning of each set of numbers resulting in incorrect data entry, even though a legend may be provided somewhere else—in a protocol or on the peel-off label.

INVESTIGATIONAL PRODUCTS LABELS—MISSING STRENGTH, BATCH/LOT NUMBER OR EXPIRY DATE

Missing IP strength or batch/lot number on IP container labels or included below a peel-off label is not in line with medication safety. Missing batch numbers create difficulties tracking expired products, promptly following up on expired/recalled products, including reporting actual or suspected adverse drug reaction.

The lack of expiry dates on IP containers can firstly result in dispensing expired products, affecting outcomes and data accuracy. Secondly, even if the products are not out of date, parents/caregivers feel unsure of whether it is safe to administer them or not, and finally, a lack of expiry date is confusing for everyone else—CT pharmacists, PIs, CRCs, CRAs, and auditors. Likewise, expiry dates on IP containers need to be consistent, allowing effortless determination of the actual expiry. Non-standardised use of a manufacture date followed by 'use by date' or 'use within X years of manufacture date' is best avoided.

Improper product packaging for the route of administration in paediatrics also poses safety risks. For example, granules or pellets packaged in capsules but intended for sprinkling on or mixing with food. While CT pharmacists include the correct directions for use on the pharmacy dispensing labels, such as 'Sprinkle on food' and 'Do not swallow', errors still happen.

Sponsors, IP manufacturers, or third-party suppliers must make certain quantities stated on IP container labels are the same as on packing slips, in the protocol, and the pharmacy manual. Deciphering the correctness of the information is inefficient, counterproductive, and requires contacting various stakeholders for clarifications. It can disadvantage participants from receiving adequate IP supply and affect the accuracy of compliance calculations.

Investigational products in bulk supply are risky in paediatric trials. Cost versus safety must be evaluated prudently. Oral IPs in bulk containers require repackaging, leading to an increased risk of errors during treatment allocation and difficulties with IP balance checking. Counting large amounts of tablets/capsules to confirm balance correctness as a first step in identifying a potential error is not practical. It can also lead to IP contamination and undesirable temperature or moisture exposure during manipulations.

UNIQUE SAFETY RISKS: WHO MANAGES THEM?

Investigational product safety risks are unique and less likely to be encountered with commercially available medicines because safeguards such as tall man lettering (TML) and bar code scanning are yet to be introduced in clinical trials. TML is a practice of writing part of medicine's name in upper case letters to help distinguish sound alike, look alike medicines from one another to avoid medication errors. The main advantages of using standardised barcoding for clinical trials are improved participants safety, reduced number of errors and cost-savings by decreasing the time consumed for manual IP chain of custody at the clinical site level and checking/double-checking dispensing process.

Detailed, IP-specific safety practices are not yet incorporated in paediatric trial protocols. In addition, there is a lack of published, standardised medication safety guidelines and limited routine involvement and input of expert paediatric pharmacists into trial design, methodology, IP administration instructions, pharmacy information resources, and data collection tools. Thus, identifying possible medication safety threats relies on the individual CT/research pharmacist's skills and practical experience in medication safety. As a result, site CT pharmacists are compelled to incorporate local medication safety guidelines, policies, and procedures into IP management. Moreover, CT pharmacists training on trial-specific safety issues, as part of site initiation visits, continues to be performed by external non-health professionals who are not necessarily familiar or passionate about the topic. The final result is that many IPs or trial safety concerns are not addressed appropriately during SIV, nor are feasible solutions provided. In brief, clinical sites pharmacists should continue preparing local trial/IP specific risk management plans/procedures to minimise identified or potential risks to participants, clinical staff, and institutions.

Table 1 is an example of an IP safety concern and suggested solution to be followed during CT implementation by the entire site clinical team.

IP SAFETY CHALLENGES	PRACTICAL SOLUTIONS
An open label CT: no blinding requirement	Mark each IP container with colour code dots
Look alike IP packaging in three strengths	Colour code
100mg tablets	Red
50mg tablets	Blue
25mg tablets	Green

Table 1: IP safety challenge and solution

Pharmacists have professionally taken over IP safety mitigation throughout trials implementation. They are expected to follow the protocol's recommendations. However, at times, pharmacists should question the provided information or instructions. It does happen that a paediatric protocol contains information from preceding adult trials. For example, a protocol recommends a dose of X mg/kg to a maximum of 1.5 mL administered subcutaneously. The logical question is whether 1.5 mL an appropriate volume for a young child? With subcutaneous injection, the medicine is injected into the fatty layer just below the skin, and those injections can cause stress, anxiety, and pain in children. It often leaves them apprehensive about receiving future injections or even becoming non-compliant with medical care. This route of administration is not appropriate for large volumes as a single injection, but an IP dose can be divided and administered by two jabs.

CT pharmacists' knowledge, skills, and experience to spot and identify safety concerns and take preventative measures are crucial. Experienced paediatric pharmacists are the best-versed health professionals to lead IP safety initiatives.

LESSONS LEARNED:

- Different IPs present different safety concerns and challenges with handling, dispensing, preparation, and administration.
- Each medication safety challenge requires a specific solution to achieve the desired benefit, thus 'one size does not fit all'.
- Best practice is to measure the benefits of implemented solutions and track the outcomes.

INCREASED SAFETY RISKS—EXAMPLES

Medication safety risks are higher with sponsors conducting more than one trial simultaneously with look alike investigational products in different strengths for different age groups. For example, siblings with the same condition were permitted to participate concurrently in two separate, double-blinded trials on the safety and efficacy of the same IP in two different age groups. The IPs for both trials were look alike, and the names/numbers were nearly the same, except for the last digits. Additionally, the IP was in two strengths, and the strength on IP container labels was hidden under a peel-off label. The two CTs were far beyond unsafe—they were dangerous.

What can be done to prevent IP mix-ups at home and increase participant safety?

In practice, increased risk of dispensing errors by pharmacists and administration errors by parents/caregivers at home can happen when IP checking relies on a single identifier, for example, a six-digit kit number in the smallest possible font.

Better safeguards are required instead of contingent on the on-site CT pharmacist initiatives when safety is compromised on multiple levels. To minimise the chance of errors at home by parents/caregivers, we used different colour coded, self-adhesive dots to mark the IP for siblings. Such mediocre solutions are not practical or suitable for solving twenty-first-century problems. Collaboration with pharmacists can formulate more appropriate solutions, such as different coloured packs or sizes for each trial and optimised labels designed for font contrasts, legibility, and layout.

Another example of imposed unsafe practice was a protocol requiring six months of dispensing followed by monthly off-site blood tests and phone dose adjustments, determined by the test results to which CT pharmacists would have no access.

It is inappropriate to provide participants with IP containers labelled with administration instructions to 'Take X tablets'; however, in a month or two, their IP doses may be changed over the phone. There is no guarantee that an incorrect dose would not be administered, as per the original label instructions. This protocol required unsafe dispensing frequency and introduced discrepancies between actual doses and administration instructions on IP containers.

The lesson learned is that medication safety management and mitigation should be a shared responsibility of all shareholders involved, rather than over-reliance on the CT pharmacists.

Outsourcing pharmacist expertise and working collaboratively towards devising preventative strategies and using more effective systems supporting medication safety is not beyond the realm of possibility.

PRESCRIBING ERROR PREVENTION

Knowing that paediatric IP prescribing and dispensing requires greater vigilance, how can we balance safe practice supporting participant well-being and providing prompt, value-added, and efficient services?

Research shows that 9.4 per cent of medication errors happen during prescribing. The answer to 'How we can reduce the chances of IP prescribing errors?' is by creating CT- customised prescription (Rx) aligned with medication safety principles.

CT prescription must comply with legislation acts and regulations and institutional policies. It must be written clearly and in compliance with the trial protocol. A physician's name and signature are required on each Rx.

Currently, trial prescriptions are created by site CT pharmacists. Some sponsors and CROs have attempted to provide their own versions. Still, they are frequently non-compliant with local legislation, policies, and practice, or incorrect and not capturing necessary information, or appearing confusing, impractical, and unacceptable for use. How to create a trial-specific prescription capturing all essential information, as per protocol, aligned with medication safety principles and yet is easy to use is described in detail in Chapter 8 under 'New Clinical Trial Set Up'.

ACCEPTABLE TERMS AND ABBREVIATIONS

The use of error-prone abbreviations, terminology, and dose expressions is one of the major causes of medication errors. While abbreviations are considered a time-saving convenience, ambiguous and unacceptable abbreviations and IP dose expressions in protocols, pharmacy manuals, and other documents pose an increased risk and can lead to errors. Their use does not promote patient safety.

- Use of abbreviations, including Latin abbreviations that are not universally understood, must be avoided.
- Always use standard abbreviations. For example, write 'units' instead of 'U', as 'U' can be mistaken for 0 ('5 U' may be seen as '50' instead of 5 units).
- Investigational product names must not be abbreviated on the CT prescriptions.

The principles of safe terms, abbreviations, and dose expressions apply to all registered medicines, investigational products, orders, and documentation, whether printed or digitally generated.

The complete list is not included in the book, as I intend to raise awareness of its existence and importance to medication safety in paediatric clinical trials.

POOR IMPLEMENTATION OF MEDICATION SAFETY INITIATIVES

'Good judgment comes from experience and experience comes from bad judgment'.

—FRED BROOKS

A sponsor's medication safety initiative to provide participants with LOCKMED boxes for safekeeping IPs at home in family fridges was exciting and very welcomed. The boxes were stylish with an aluminium exterior and a beautiful dark velvet interior. But they were impractical because they were too bulky and unsuitable for fridge IP storing due to interior moulding. Parents did not want them, not even for other purposes, because of their size and heavy weight. A great idea was poorly implemented. Were there other, more suitable, and practical options? Certainly, fridge-appropriate boxes are produced from high-impact resistant polycarbonate. They are shatter-resistant, lightweight, portable, with a digital combination code lock and ventilation slots for safe storage of medicines in fridges and freezers up to −80°C, equivalent to −112°F.

Consulting pharmacists with appropriate expertise and experience about practicality and cost effectiveness could have prevented the flawed implementation of a good idea. As a health professional for over two decades in the public healthcare sector, I am well acquainted with the ongoing growth in healthcare expenditure and effective cost containment. Therefore, *Evolving the Dinosaur* is aligned with evidence-based principles and pharmacoeconomic and practicality considerations to achieve the best possible safety outcomes with limited resources.

Another example of a poorly executed safety initiative was the provision of TempAlert devices for home temperature monitoring of fridge-stored IPs. Sponsor-initiated safety measures are a pleasant surprise because someone else from the outside thought about it.

But if poor quality or unreliable devices are considered, it is seen as another ineffective initiative and an unjustifiable expense.

The temperature monitoring devices displayed 'OK' on their tiny screens for weeks and months, regardless of temperature changes from ambient to refrigeration and back to ambient. Some device screens randomly went black. What did a blank screen mean? I could not find information about it, and none was provided. The protocol instructions were clear: if a tag alert does not show OK, do not use the product. I did some experiments with devices returned by participants. The OK sign was disappearing randomly on some devices for days, on others for weeks, but the majority were OK forever, no matter what.

Were they reliable? No one knew. Was it a good idea to have continuous temperature monitoring at home? Yes—it was brilliant! Could it have been implemented better? Yes, with reusable and downloadable devices. Acquisition cost would have been higher, but what is the price of participants omitting doses, affecting the data, and discarding tens of hundreds of vials without being sure whether the IP was compromised, or the devices were malfunctional?

EXCIPIENTS IN PAEDIATRIC FORMULATIONS

Excipients or additives are used in pharmaceutical formulations to enhance solubility or stability, as flavouring agents, preservatives, sweeteners, and for taste masking or tablet compaction. Their use should be considered carefully, as they may cause adverse effects in infants and children. Commonly, it is assumed that because they are inert and pharmacologically inactive, they are safe. However, not all excipients used in adult medications are suitable for the paediatric population. Neonates, infants, and children may not be able to metabolise or eliminate them in the same way and rate comparing to adults due to the immaturity of their hepatic and renal systems.

Paediatric dosing is weight-based; thus, neonates, infants, and young children can be exposed to a higher amount than recommended for adults. Listing the excipient names and amounts on IP labels or in IP handling manuals would allow PIs and CT pharmacists to assess safety limits for individual trial participants when and if required. Currently, the names of excipients may be listed, but the amounts are rarely provided.

The topic of excipient use in paediatric medicinal products and their effect is not within the scope of this book. However, I want to present some basic information on the most frequently used excipients: gelatine, artificial sweeteners, colouring agents, solvents, preservatives, castor oil, and arachis (peanut) oil.

GELATINE

Gelatine is derived from animal products, which understandably is *concern for vegetarians, vegans, and people of specific faiths.* CT pharmacists frequently deal with such queries. The use of gelatine is relatively common in capsules, and it certainly generates lots of questions, whether it is kosher or made from fish. If information is not provided, obviously, we cannot answer the queries.

ARTIFICIAL SWEETENERS

Aspartame and saccharin are used to enhance palatability or to disguise unpleasant taste. They are undesirable in children with certain disorders. For example, children with phenylketonuria must avoid aspartame.

Glucose and sucrose are also sweeteners, and their use in oral medications can contribute to obesity and tooth decay, especially if administered at bedtime.

Carbohydrate content must be accounted for and minimised for children on a ketogenic diet (a high-fat, low-carbohydrate, and restricted protein diet, helpful in patients with refractory seizures).

COLOURING AGENTS

They convey distinctive appearance to pharmaceutical dosage forms, improve acceptability to patients, and help consumers distinguish non-prescription from prescription medications. The use of colouring agents can increase the stability of light-sensitive active ingredients in tablets and capsules. Some synthetic dyes may negatively affect young children. For example, tartrazine has been associated with hypersensitivity and behavioural disturbances in some children.

SOLVENTS

Paediatric formulations containing ethanol, used as a solvent, could lead to intoxication, central nervous system effects, and hypoglycaemia. Also, it can cause a disulfiram-like reaction when given in combination with certain medications (e.g., metronidazole). If ethanol is present in investigational formulations, full disclosure of its presence and concentration is essential.

Propylene glycol (PG) is a commonly used solvent in oral, intravenous, and topical pharmaceutical products. It is generally safe, but when used in high doses or for prolonged periods, adverse effects such as central nervous system toxicity, hyperosmolarity, cardiac arrhythmia, seizures, and lactic acidosis have been reported. Caution should be exercised with medications containing PG, especially in infants.

Sorbitol—often used as a humectant, plasticiser, and sweetening agent—can cause diarrhea, abdominal pain, and flatulence when given in excess amounts.

PRESERVATIVES

Benzyl alcohol is used as a preservative, and it has been related to gasping syndrome (seizures, metabolic acidosis, renal/hepatic abnormalities, cardiovascular collapse, including death) in neonates. Benzoic acid / sodium benzoate can cause jaundice, displace bilirubin from albumin, and potentially cause kernicterus in neonates.

CASTOR OIL AND ARACHIS (PEANUT) OIL

Used as solubilizing agents, castor oil and arachis (peanut) oil, can cause anaphylactic reactions.

The lack of safety and toxicity data on some of the frequently used excipients is a well-documented hurdle in paediatric formulation development. A current lack of comprehensive excipient risk assessments in paediatrics, coupled with excipient innovation, and development of new novel ones may further widen the gap between deficiency of evidence supporting and opposing their use in children.

It would be beneficial if the content of excipients in investigational formulations are identified, itemised, quantitatively specified, and provided together with safety limits, if available.

TIPS FOR ADMINISTRATING INVESTIGATIONAL PRODUCTS TO INFANTS AND CHILDREN

Medication compliance in paediatric patients is affected by many factors, such as age, ease of administration, taste, smell, formulation type, time of administration, family lifestyle and dynamics, formulation suitability for the child/parents/caregivers, and the provision of clear spoken or written information.

Administration of IPs to infants and children follows the exact instructions provided in the protocol. Comprehensive training on IP administration for trial participants' parents and caregivers is fundamental for correct dosing and compliance. Contradictory or confusing information and administration instructions hinder compliance and should be avoided at any cost.

My personal experience is that when participants/parents/guardians are provided with unambiguous and well-illustrated instructions for home administration of IPs, they feel confident about what, how much, when, and how to, which leads to higher compliance. In addition, compliance is enhanced by visual demonstrations, understanding, and addressing parents' apprehension or fears to help them feel safe and connected.

Patient information leaflets continue to be written at a level that is difficult to understand. Research reveals that only 30 per cent of caregivers can calculate and measure the correct dose of paracetamol when provided with manufacturer packaging and measuring devices.[20] The lesson learned is that parents need substantial support with managing medicine administration at home—irrespective of being registered or investigational.

One of the most frequent queries CT pharmacists encounter

by parents is about IPs' interactions with milk and food, items standardly consumed by children. Therefore, paediatric protocols and pharmacy manuals must specify if oral IPs can be given pre/post milk, at the very least.

INVESTIGATIONAL PRODUCTS FOR ORAL ADMINISTRATION

Even though some sponsors have started offering swallowability tests to establish tablet or capsule size appropriateness before enrolling participants, I would like to address a few practical points.

The age at which a child can learn to swallow tablets and capsules varies, but suitable candidates should be at least four years of age, cooperative, and motivated to learn new skills. Training and support from healthcare professionals and parents/caregivers are equally important. A simple method to start is cutting gummy bears into small pieces and allowing the child to swallow each with water. As the child gets better, we may gradually increase the cut sizes to match the tablet or capsule they need to take.

The advantages of using liquid formulations in children are that they are ready to use and easy to measure doses. The disadvantages are higher production costs, stability issues, and shorter shelf life than solid forms. Also, liquid formulations are linked to excipients-related allergic reactions, problems with ingredients used as co-solvents (ethanol, sorbitol), and are not practical to carry around.

Advantages of using tablets and capsules are that they are easy to carry, generally have a long expiry, and lower production cost than liquids. Their disadvantages are administration difficulties and the need for cutting, crushing, or opening capsules and tablets, which may not always be an appropriate manipulation.

Dispersible tablets are suitable for infants and children because they are easy to manipulate and administer.

CAUTION with dispersing immunosuppressive or teratogenic IPs in spoons to avoid spilling, contamination, and parent/caregiver exposure. The best practice is to provide step-by-step instructions for dose preparation in an oral syringe.

An example of instructions for dispersing IP (tablets) in an oral syringe is provided in the appendix. The template can be modified as required.

INVESTIGATIONAL PRODUCTS FOR INTRAVENOUS (IV) AND INTRAMUSCULAR (IM) ADMINISTRATION

Children generally do not like needles. The ability to accurately measure small volumes injections is of particular importance. Active ingredient concentration appropriateness is crucial to avoid further manipulations or dilutions. If dilution is required, suitable diluents, final concentration, and the final product's shelf life, including the rate of administration, must be specified.

Intramuscular (IM) administration in children is painful due to their small muscle mass and should generally be avoided. Neonates have poorly perfused muscles, and thus, IM administration rarely provides adequate therapeutic levels, as the medicine remains in the muscle for prolonged periods.

Injection volumes should be small and not exceed 1 mL at a single site. Hospital guidelines limit the volume to 0.5 mL per site for newborns and small infants, 1 mL per single site for small children, and 2 mL per site in older, school-age children with a well-developed muscle mass to tolerate injection.

The addition of a local inaesthetic may reduce the incidence and duration of pain, but only if appropriate. Consideration should be given to the maximum concentration of a reconstituted IP vial (minimum volume of diluent) to make the final administration volume as small as possible.

HOW TO MASK UNPLEASANT TASTE

IPs should never be mixed with milk in feeding bottles or with large quantities of food because there is no guarantee the contents of the whole bottle or food will be consumed by the child, meaning they will take an unknown proportion of the dose. Additional concerns are milk-IP or food-IP interactions, including the possibility of IPs unpleasantly affecting the milk or food taste, resulting in future refusal of these items. A small amount of food (e.g., on a teaspoon) is the preferable method to disguise the taste while ensuring the entire dose is taken.

Although the contents of capsules can be sprinkled over food, appropriate precautions should be taken to avoid exposing the person preparing and administering the doses. Note that it may be inappropriate for pregnant women to manipulate teratogenic products.

An unpleasant aftertaste can be disguised by giving the child their favourite food or drink immediately after a dose if permitted by the trial protocol.

Suggested foods to disguise the taste, if not on the trial's prohibited food list, are:

- Spoonful of yogurt
- Spoonful of soft food like mashed pumpkin or apple puree

- Ice cream toppings: strawberry or chocolate
- Spoonful of honey

CAUTION! Children under the age of twelve months are at risk of infant botulism if they consume honey.

Sponsors are encouraged to provide instructions about IP administration via nasogastric (NG) feeding tubes. Children on NG feeding should take the IPs by mouth when and if possible. If not, and in the absence of specific administration instructions, the usual practice is to stop the enteral feeds before the dose is given. The tubes are flushed well with water before and after IP administration. Stopping enteral feeding for a certain period before and after doses may be recommended if enteral feeds reduce IP absorption.

INVESTIGATIONAL PRODUCTS ADHERENCE

Participant adherence, also known as compliance, is an essential part of every clinical trial. IP non-compliance in paediatric trials is a complex, multilayered problem involving the participants and their parents/caregivers/family members.

'Drugs don't work in patients who don't take them'.

—C. EVERETT KOOP, MD, US SURGEON GENERAL, 1985

Investigational products' safety and effectiveness cannot be assessed if they are not taken. Statistically, medication adherence rates in paediatric patients are variable and range from 11 to 93 per cent. However, even chronic disease sufferers, such as those with juvenile rheumatoid arthritis, post organ transplant, cancer, and epilepsy patients, only have medication compliance rates between 50 to 60 per cent.[21]

What are the reasons for non-compliance?

A child's age plays a significant role, as infants and children are dependent on their parents/caregivers to give them the IPs. That changes as they grow up and become more responsible over their treatment(s) and better understand their disease. Still, it does not necessarily lead to improved compliance. Driven by the desire to appear just like everyone else, they may not take their IPs during sleepovers at friends' houses because of the stigma of taking medicines or being embarrassed to disclose personal health issues. In addition, IPs associated with cosmetic side effects, such as weight gain or acne, have shown a low compliance rate because these side effects have an emotional and body image impact.

Sociocultural reasons affecting compliance are related to insufficient information about the disease and the treatment or not understanding them. For example, non-English speaking trial participants and their families may have language barriers.

Currently, sponsors are providing interpreters to cover the physician's part of a clinical visit. However, a more appropriate option would be covering the entire visit or at least the first IPs counselling by a CT pharmacist.

The family structure, parental attitude towards the disease and treatment, and the interpersonal relationships between the family members are also important. Research and practice concur that family conflict relations are associated with unsatisfactory compliance rates. Conversely, a family's understanding of their child's condition and support and concern about the treatment's safety and efficacy are linked to higher compliance rates.

In paediatrics, medicines adherence is achieved by focussing on the participants and their parents or caregivers. Therefore, the provision of precise and well-illustrated administration instructions or demonstration is essential.

IPs' dosing and administration schedules are fundamental for compliance. Midday doses present difficulties for school children, leading to missed doses. Compliance rates decrease as the dose administration frequency increases, and commonly increase at the beginning of the trial rather than towards the end.

Also, children may refuse to take IPs due to taste, smell, aftertaste, or texture.

Practice proven strategies and interventions:

- Participant and family education to understand their child's disease, the CT, and the role of IPs encourages compliance.
- CT/research pharmacists are the most appropriate health professionals to tackle IP compliance issues. They are at the forefront of patient care and know-how to build a trust-based relationship with patients and their families, address potential compliance issues, and offer customised solutions.
- Understanding why poor compliance or why specific doses are missed helps when working out a personalised solution. In some instances, children may like to be involved with their therapy if probed and engaged appropriately.

As a clinical pharmacist, I had renal transplant patients who prevented medication errors upon hospital admissions. I had taught them what amount of each liquid medicine and how many tablets of different colours or shapes they take. I had led them to question their medication if handed something different by a nurse or anyone else looking after them. As a result, the kids were proud of knowing their medicines and doses and did not hesitate to show it.

The family lifestyle and the number of caregivers involved usually reveal possible compliance issues or actions required. Often, what parents and caregivers need is a health professional who can offer understanding and reassurance and address their fears and concerns.

Paediatric pharmacists know how to engage children playfully by using stuffed animals and speaking in simple terms. However, not every toddler will be receptive, so do not forget to assess the child's comfort level with strangers.

In conclusion, for increased compliance rates across clinical sites, coaching and IPs counselling standardisation are critical. Currently, the practice is widely variable, depending on the principal investigator's preferences. Often, participant counselling is delegated to CRCs who may or may not be health professionals with paediatric experience. While each professional claims to be doing what is best for the patient, pharmacists continue to be the most suitable professionals to counsel patients and families on the IP's role, accurate dosing and administration, and recording.

HOW TO IMPROVE INVESTIGATIONAL PRODUCTS ADHERENCE

Technology promoted IP administration, such as smartphone apps and calendars, are convenient reminders of the dosing schedules (for example, GlowCaps for medicine bottles).

Linking IP administration times with daily living activities is helpful.

To promote IP adherence in a trial, site pharmacists or externally outsourced consultant pharmacists can combine expertise with drug development teams to identify simpler IP regimens with easier administration schedules to decrease the dosing burden placed on parents and caregivers.

Children can take their medication first thing in the morning, after school, and at bedtime, if this approach works for the child's condition, for the parents, and is aligned with the trial protocol.

Improving or masking the taste of medicines can have a positive effect on compliance. Note: these suggestions can only be used when permitted by trial protocols.

- Giving ice cubes or popsicles to children before a medicine may numb taste buds and mask unpleasant taste.
- Acidic juices such as orange juice can be used to dissipate an unpleasant aftertaste.
- Salty tasting medication can be concealed by butterscotch, cinnamon, or peanut butter.
- Chocolate, coffee flavouring, or liquorice can be used to conceal bitterness.
- Chilled medication may be more acceptable, but only if the IPs are stable at refrigerated temperatures.
- Larger volumes of oral liquid formulations are better avoided in children, regardless of the taste. In practice, general unwillingness to take large volumes has been observed.

CAUTION! Mixing IPs with food or juice should be avoided due to interactions and stability issues.

Practical solutions for IP adherence are:

- Individualised counselling
- Simplified dosing regimens
- Use of technology
- Tactics to improve or mask taste/aftertaste

LESSONS LEARNED:

- Changes in IP formulations and/or dosage regimen during trial implementation must be promptly communicated directly to site CT pharmacists, as they may lead to new and unexpected administration and safety challenges.
- IP dosing frequency that coincides with the family/child's lifestyle leads to improved compliance rates.
- IP interactions with milk and food, typical for children, should be addressed in trial protocols, pharmacy manuals, and if oral IPs can be given pre/post milk, at the very least.
- Excipients are not inert agents just because they lack pharmacological action.
- Children are NOT small adults.
- They are at increased risk of medication errors and adverse drug reactions.
- If unsure, seek advice!

PART TWO

The Measurement Plan

WITH ADHERENCE TO LEGISLATION, CLINICAL TRIAL PROTOCOL, INSTITUTIONAL RESEARCH GOVERNANCE FRAMEWORK, AND PHARMACOVIGILANCE

'If you aren't measuring the right things to begin with, you're not going to get better results by measuring them more accurately'.

—UNKNOWN

CHAPTER FIVE

What to Measure

PAEDIATRIC CLINICAL TRIAL SERVICE BASELINE ASSESSMENT AND MEASUREMENT

'If you don't like how things are, change it. You are not a tree'.

—JIM ROHN

SERVICE BENCHMARKING

Benchmarking in health is used to improve efficiency, quality of care, patient safety, and satisfaction. Each of these individually or collectively contribute towards *Evolving the Dinosaur*; my next step was to apply it in practice.

Benchmarking is a process of measuring the performance of products, services, or processes against those considered the best in the industry or of a high, recognisable standard. The two most frequently used types in healthcare are internal and external benchmarking. Measured dimensions typically are quality, time, and cost.

I decided to start with external comparative benchmarking of practices and service performance by contacting pharmacy CT services in three Australian tertiary paediatric hospitals with a specially created questionnaire for data collection. The idea was to gather data from other paediatric sites for comparison. Unfortunately, the project failed for the following reasons: different scope of service, service funding, staffing, and practices—all hindering comparative benchmarking. The next logical step was to conduct a CT service baseline performance, financial and scope evaluation, and identify appropriate metrics due to the lack of standardised key performance indicators (KPIs) for paediatric pharmacy clinical trial services or guidance about suitable metrics for data collection.

KEY PERFORMANCE INDICATORS AND METRICS

KPIs and metrics explained: The similarities between the two are that they are quantifiable or measurable values, and both must be very well defined. The key difference is that all KPIs are metrics, but not all metrics are KPIs.

So, while KPIs reflect CT pharmacy service objectives and how successful we are in accomplishing them, metrics reflect how successful our actions are to achieve the KPIs. In other words, KPIs define a set of values against which the metrics are measured. Guided by the saying that we 'cannot improve what we cannot measure' and 'what gets measured, gets done', I moved on with identifying metrics, collecting data, and establishing an accurate service status.

Note: CT service may have many KPIs, but it is crucial to choose the ones that drive it forward.

My initial assessment showed the CT service failed to keep pace with the increasing demands without compromising service scope and quality. It required multifaceted and rapid change management, which would not have happened in a timely fashion had I gone through the chain of command. Senior pharmacy management would have had difficulties identifying what urgent service needs are and what changes are required to formulate prompt strategies and solutions. Therefore, it is imperative in those fast-evolving areas of the pharmacy that the decision-making authority is assigned to whoever manages the service to act as facilitators of the most advantageous changes. Higher commitment is better sustained when employees feel ownership.

I carried out the change management as *an emergent change*, meaning I placed less weight on extensive planning and projections and focused on the pressing service needs to operate more efficiently and shift its boundaries and interactions. Unlike planned change, which is usually top-down, my approach was bottom-up.

The change management framework implementation included:

1. Measuring CT service scope, operational, and financial performance.
2. Analysing the data.
3. Implementing the data-guided changes through a safe course of actions.

The immediate CT service requirements were to re-establish its professional identity and place among the internal and external stakeholders, institute more effective cross-functional communication, collaboration, workflows streamlining, and to map out scaling strategies to generate consistent trials/participants volume and revenue growth.

Building bridges with relevant stakeholders offered multiple benefits throughout the change implementation, ranging from avoiding misunderstandings and resistance to gaining engagement and commitment. I could not have succeeded without an effective exchange of information, consultations, involvement, and radical, real-time collaboration for goals and resources alignment.

The change management framework also included work processes mapping to identify the necessity for further improvements. In addition, workflow analysis and developing a logical sequence of the trial's operational activities helped clarify what changes were consistent with the research teams and pharmacy CT service goals.

Generally, education and training are fundamental parts of the change management process. However, the process of rebuilding the clinical trials/research as a service involved health professionals who already had established skill sets, expertise, and experiences. Thus, establishing transparent, two-way communication avenues to vent frustrations, applaud what is working, and seamlessly change what is not, proved to be more authentic and practical than education and training. It worked out well.

LESSONS LEARNED:

- Map out where the CT service going, why and how to get there.
- Set priorities according to pressing needs and create a change management plan.

- Gain other clinical research stakeholder engagement and commitment.
- Implement change.
- Reinforce it by continuing communication, coordination, and cooperation.
- Sustain it.

CT/research service performance is measured mainly by numbers, financial performance is inherently tied to the dollar sign, and service scope by the range of services provided (essential versus comprehensive). Other practical dimensions in clinical trials measure the time taken to complete a task, time per pharmacist hourly rate in dollars, and cost per item. Later in Chapter 6 and 7, I elaborate on each one in the context of trial feasibility assessment and budgeting for trial-related pharmacy services.

MEASURING OPERATIONAL PERFORMANCE

Why did I have to measure the CT service operational performance? Because it had been overcommitted, with questionable capabilities to deliver end-to-end, quality services. Thus, it was essential to establish a service performance baseline to guide future planning and staffing requirements. I followed Peter Drucker quote: 'What gets measured, gets managed'.

The metrics we can use depend on the questions we are trying to answer. As the proverb goes: 'measure what you treasure'.

Examples of metrics I used to attain meaningful data:

- Total number of active CTs—internal (investigator-driven) and external (pharma sponsored)
- Number of enrolled participants per trial

- Number of clinical visits, requiring IP dispensing per participant, per trial
- Number of IP items dispensed per visit
- Number of months' supply per visit
- Number of CTs by stage of *implementation—recently started versus soon to close out. I used time* in months to trial completion as the most practical metric
- Number of CTs by the degree of complexity: simple, medium, and complex
- Number of future participant enrolment for trials still open for enrolment
- Number of trials in the pipeline to start
- Time in minutes per specific trial-related tasks: dispensing, IP receiving, destruction, and so on
- CT pharmacists' time in minutes per monitoring visit per trial
- Number of pharmacists' interventions per trial per month
- CT pharmacists' time in minutes per intervention
- Number of prevented IP errors per month
- Number of actual IP errors per month
- Number of errors on logs per monitor visit
- Number of incorrect accountability entries of returned IPs requiring corrections per monitor visit
- Number of successful budgets completed per unit time

I focused on measuring only those that provided adequate data to support improvements, starting with the most urgent and vital from the many possible questions and metrics.

The KPIs against which the metrics were measured are as follows:

1. **Participants' Wait Time:** Calculated by the average amount

of time a participant was waiting for IP dispensing. I used the time a prescription was handed in and completed/ready to be handed out, measured in time units (minutes).

2. **CT Pharmacy Monitoring Visit Duration:** Calculated by the average amount of time a CRA spends in pharmacy CT service, measured in time units (minutes).
3. **CT Pharmacist to Participants Ratio:** Denotes staff capacity. For example, a low pharmacist-to-patient ratio indicates high workloads, affecting the quality of care, expressed in numbers.
4. **Communication Events Between CT Pharmacist and PI/CRCs:** Determines the communication frequency between CT pharmacist and PI/CRC per participant visit, measured by a number of documented communication events.

Note: the duration of communication was not recorded or accounted for, as it was not practical. Regular communication led to expeditious services and participant/parent satisfaction.

5. **Participant Satisfaction:** Satisfaction levels were considered high when waiting time for IP supply reduced or eliminated. Customer satisfaction is related to the provision of timely, efficient, and patient-centred healthcare services. I used a short, four-question survey administered by the research coordinators.
6. **Number of Dispensing Error Events:** Measured by the number of errors made by CT pharmacists. Assessment of the reasons leading to an error is paramount for future preventative actions. Nil errors also are linked to employee effectiveness.
7. **Number of Prevented IP Error Events:** Measured by the number of prevented errors that may have led to participant's harm. The number is indicative of how safe a CT pharmacists' practice is.

Using real-time data allowed prompt implementation of practice and process changes. For example, reducing monitoring visit duration by an average of thirty minutes (for simple CTs) and forty-five minutes (for complex) per visit. In addition, the implemented changes in practice, led to a significant reduction of errors on logs and incorrectly recorded events.

I am proud that in a short time, the CT service not only achieved the targeted improvements, but time proved that they were sustainable.

Next, I explore what metrics we can use to measure financial performance.

MEASURING FINANCIAL PERFORMANCE

Measuring financial performance is fundamental for self-funded pharmacy CT services' sustainability and future scaling and growth to support a greater number of CTs.

Examples of metrics I used are as follows:

- Number of active CTs times dollar value per trial (pharmacy fees as per clinical trial agreement)
- Number of dispensed items times dollar value per month supply or participant visit

For a baseline financial assessment, I examined whether the pharmacy trial-related services fees were relevant or in need of an adjustment. Generally, it depends on when the trial agreement was last negotiated and executed. I also looked at the fee appropriateness for trial complexity and the actual time consumed per key tasks.

CT complexity is arbitrary, and it has been a point of ongoing difference of opinion between pharmacists and sponsors or their delegates during budgeting. In the absence of a standardised definition, for simplicity and transparency, I used the following descriptions:

- Simple trial requires straightforward IP management.
- A medium complex trial requires additional time for specific tasks beyond IP receiving, dispensing, accountability of returns and recording.
- A complex trial requires IP manufacturing or further aseptic/non-aseptic manipulation of the original packaging or additional unusual handling. A significant difference between adult and paediatric CTs is the practice of double-checking and signing the correctness of IP doses, strength, and calculations.

Finally, I looked at any other tasks performed that may have been unknown during pharmacy budget preparation and not considered.

Once I set my database up with the targeted metrics and included the pharmacy fees per CT agreement, it ended up being quite a straightforward analysis to obtain relevant reports or estimate the service's future financial outlook.

I used the initial service financial performance to guide the budgeting improvements required for funding additional staff and service sustainability.

SCOPE OF SERVICE EVALUATION

Does the pharmacy CT service provide basic or comprehensive services?

Basic trial services include:

- CT initiation
- IP inventory management and control
- Accountability
- Storage
- Temperature monitoring
- CT prescription creation
- Dispensing
- Maintenance of IP disposal records, destruction, or return
- CT closeout

Comprehensive, end-to-end CT service incorporates all the above, in addition to trial budgeting, regular billing for pharmacy services, and attending and actively participating in interdisciplinary team meetings and scientific committee/EC/IRB.

The CT service I inherited had a fascinating history—its scope had changed from end to end to basic over three to four years. Discounting the reasons for the adverse change, I wanted to rebuild it, make it self-sustainable, and give it the capability to grow organically.

I am passionate about CT pharmacists being adept in assessing the scope of their services in this exponentially growing area. The line between base and comprehensive CT service provision is not static and changes rapidly, similarly to the sudden growth of a medium-sized CT service to a large one.

Pharmacists' managed CT services are in desperate need of current, actual data and time tracked trial-related tasks and duties for future standardisation and automation.

PHARMACY FOLDERS ASSESSMENT

Before discussing the initial assessment of pharmacy CT folders, I would like to clarify that for this book, a basic definition of an *assessment* is 'the process of gathering and fashioning data into an interpretable form for decision making' and *measurement* is 'the action of measuring the identified metrics'.

Why is self-assessment essential? Firstly, proper documentation is critical to the success of a clinical trial, and every aspect must be documented to obtain valuable data. GCP guidelines list the essential documents (ICH GCP E6 Section 8) that the sites must maintain for every clinical trial. Therefore, no matter how differently pharmacy CT units operate, the process of essential documentation assessments or self-assessments and verification by the sponsors representative remains the same.

Secondly, the pharmacy trial-related tasks are connected to the clinical research objectives. For example, an increase in IP accountability log accuracy led to decreased monitoring visits durations and increased CRAs satisfaction.

Well-organised pharmacy folders are a direct reflection of a pharmacist's organisational skills, the service itself and the clinical site.

A well-managed CT unit coupled with accurate and complete paperwork/data collection logs is referred to as a 'pleasure to work with' and foster enhanced reputation and creditability. The pharmacy CT service image and creditability are beneficial for both future budget negotiations with the same sponsors and as a measure of customer satisfaction. As Victoria Dennis said, 'Our reputation precedes us'. Intriguingly, my personal experience had been long-established by research papers, showing that reputation is the major independent variable with a significant relationship with customer satisfaction and loyalty.[22]

WHAT TO LOOK FOR

Pharmacy trial folder contents are relatively standard, but my initial assessment was focused on the CT pharmacists'-created dispensing summaries, prescriptions, IP accountability logs (IPALs), shipping documentation, management of returned IPs by participants, and pharmacy staff training and delegation logs.

TRIAL-SPECIFIC DISPENSING SUMMARIES

Site pharmacists' created trial-specific dispensing summaries serve as a quick guide.

I started the preliminary assessment by finding the answers to the following questions:

- Are dispensing summaries available?
- Do they appear current and correct?
- Is there a version control?
- How is it tracked?
- Who creates them?
- Who updates them and when? Immediately after each protocol amendment approval or when time permits?
- How EC/IRB approved trial protocols and amendments are delivered to the pharmacy CT service? What institutional

policy/procedures are in place to govern trial documentation management?
- Is the current practice efficient?
- Are the dispensing summaries required for training other pharmacy staff?
- Are they actually used?

My initial assessment uncovered that the dispensing summaries were created at some stage by someone who was no longer working in the area. The summaries appeared to be inaccurate and not in line with the latest protocol amendments. There was no version control and no one accountable for their accuracy and updates. Therefore, I decided not to use them but instead rely on the latest approved protocols and pharmacy manuals. While reading the pharmacy resources, I marked relevant, important information on pages with multicoloured stickers for quick future reference. It was not an ideal solution, but good enough under the circumstances. It worked for me at the time. Large CT units may consider creating an SOP for preparing dispensing summaries, if not already existing, to drive internal standardisation across trials.

CLINICAL TRIAL CUSTOMISED PRESCRIPTION (RX)

Similarly to the initial assessment of the dispensing summaries, I started by questioning the trial Rx format accuracy and legality with applicable laws, regulations, and standards.

Example questions for assessment:

- Is there a prescription version control?
- Is the newest version currently used for each visit?
- How are the dispensed prescriptions filed? Is the most

functional filing in place? How easy is it to find Rx-related information?
- Are the prescriptions filed by date of dispensing, per participant visit, or per participant's ID number?

What worked best at the time was to keep each participant's prescriptions together with the interactive response technology IP assignments printouts plus/minus dose calculation or preparation sheets, if applicable, and the participant's accountability logs together.

The benefits were: they appeared neat and organised, convenient to keep track of participants visits, and were practical and time-saving solution for CRAs and auditors.

ASSESSMENT OF IP ACCOUNTABILITY LOGS AND RECORDKEEPING

Example questions for an IP accountability logs (IPALs) assessment:

- How many logs need to be completed per participant for each trial?
- What entries are required?
- Is there a need for improvement?
- If yes, what is the issue, and how could it be rectified?

Factors contributing to recording omissions on logs are the lack of technological advances and excessive manual entries on multiple logs. For example, a trial may require the completion of logs for different IP strengths, logs for the comparators, participant enrolment logs, and ancillary item logs.

Change of IP dispensing workflow with integrated log completion resulted in a reduction in both entry omissions and errors.

Sponsors/CROs usually provide the IPALs. Unfortunately, both paper and electronic ones can be inappropriate if they lack columns for documenting/entering required transactions. What is the solution? CT pharmacists create their own, then seek approval for use from the sponsors/their delegate. Then sponsors/CROs update their accountability logs, and pharmacists are trained on how to use them. Can we skip some unnecessary steps? Yes, by including the right people to create the right tools and standardise the data collection tools across all clinical sites.

SHIPPING RECORDS ASSESSMENT

For the IPs' shipping records documentation assessment, I looked at their completeness/missing paperwork, recording, and the filing process.

- Are they recorded correctly?
- Are they filed by invoice/packing slip numbers or by date of receipt?
- Is any improvement required?

The CT monitors and auditors inspect shipping record documentation, thus, keeping each shipment's paperwork together (in a separate plastic sleeve) proved to be an efficient and practical approach for their long-term management. A small change made the pharmacy folders well organised, reduced monitor/auditor verification time during inspections, and allowed prompt retrieval of information when required.

MANAGEMENT OF RETURNED INVESTIGATIONAL PRODUCTS ASSESSMENT

Example questions for assessment of how returned IPs are managed

1. What is the CT service's usual practice?
2. Are returned IPs accounted for immediately, the same day or when time permits?
3. Are there dedicated areas for IP returns, separating those already accounted for and documented versus those that are not?
4. On how many logs are returned IPs recorded?
5. Are there unfilled spots on the logs? What is the reason? Are those IPs not processed yet or not returned by a participant?
6. Are there many corrections on the logs? If not, what is nature—incorrect IP counting, measuring, or something else? Are the corrections signed/dated?

Often, CT pharmacists are too busy to perform accountability of returns immediately. However, they can be placed in a clear plastic Ziplock bag, endorsed with the participant's ID, visit number, and date of return before being placed in a dedicated area for processing when time permits. The benefits are that entries are more accurate when counting is performed and monitors take less time for their reconciliation. I was pleasantly surprised when the same sponsor voluntary provided plastic Ziplock bags for participant returns for their second and third trial with our site. It worked like a charm!

WORKFLOW STREAMLINING AND MEASURING PERFORMANCE

Workflow is a sequence of tasks or actions that need to be completed consecutively. It is the way work gets done. For example, during a clinical visit, the tests and procedures are in sequence. If we know the order—who does what and approximately when—we can have a clear understanding of the workflow and fit the IP dispensing within the visit cycle instead of at the end of it, and eliminate participants' wait time for pharmacy services.

Workflow streamlining requires measuring its performance post-implementation to identify problems and bottlenecks needing further modification or fine-tuning. Almost always, *the adjustments are upfront* because each clinical visit differs in length, variety of tests and procedures.

Streamlining workflow in paediatric CTs is challenging but rewarding for everyone involved once it is achieved.

Some important questions to start with are:

- What is the usual internal workflow of pharmacy CT service?
- What is the general workflow of a clinical visit?
- Can pharmacy IP dispensing fit in with the participant visits?

If a workflow is not efficient and would benefit from a redesign, what metrics can we choose for measuring its performance?

I used the duration of a participant's visit as *a lead time* and the time taken to complete pharmacy IP dispensing for the same visit as *a cycle time.*

Lead time is the time between the start and end of a participant's visit. Different visits are of various durations.

Cycle time is when a prescription is handed in and when the dispensed IPs are ready for collection. Cycle time includes the steps of dispensing and recording on logs process (internal pharmacy workflow).

Measuring and analysing both metrics helped me identify task duration and adjust the processes accordingly to meet my key objective: IP dispensing completed before the visit's end. Rather than working in order of first come, first-served, I manipulated the internal prescriptions processing flow. The visit duration and the time required to complete IP dispensing guided the order in which prescriptions were distributed. For example, IP dispensing for short visits were prioritised over IP orders for long-duration visits.)

Workflow redesign is a time-consuming task due to the specific requirements during each visit and the complexity of individual trials because workflow assessment was performed individually for each clinical visit. However, the benefits of increased efficiency, reduction in errors, data recording omissions, and keeping up CT services and tasks on schedule far outweighed the initial heavy time investment and the difficulties experienced.

Testing a newly designed workflow for a while, to give it a chance, is essential.

Knowing the participant visits upfront and including them into my planner was a more efficient way of managing site clinical visits. As each participant's visit is booked in advance, the PI and CRC knew when the participant would be in and what would be performed; it was just a matter of being included in the communication loop.

A weekly planner worked better for reconfirmed participants bookings. For clinical visits, where IP doses were independent of body weight on the day of the visit, IPs were pre-ordered, pre-dispensed, and ready for collection from the CT pharmacy. Sponsors have been receptive and supportive when a 'note to file' (NTF) or an SOP accurately describing the process was provided.

Note: the dispensed IPs were always kept safely in the pharmacy, and temperature monitored until collection.

What information was most beneficial for the pharmacy visit planner? A participant ID, visit number and duration, date and time of arrival, and the PI/SI appointment time.

To adjust the internal pharmacy CT service workflow, I have used the following steps:

- Evaluate specific process workflow.
- Streamline movement of incoming and outgoing tasks, like prescriptions, IP shipments, participant returns, and dispensed IPs.
- Implement directional workflow and look for steps stalling the flow.
- Practice if it works well. Make changes that free up time for other value-added activities.
- Review processes regularly and adjust as required.

CHAPTER SIX

New Clinical Trials

It is impossible to separate the ongoing CT service assessments, gathering and fashioning data to guide decision making from the assessments made before accepting to conduct a new trial and during the preparation to start. Therefore, I have included new CT feasibility visits, pharmacy budgeting, and internal pharmacy set up into the measurement part of the book. While these initial new trial related assessments are not actual measurements, they are captured and used for quantitative or qualitative measurements and tracking throughout the trial implementation.

IS FEASIBILITY ASSESSMENT FEASIBLE? CAN IT BE IMPROVED?

The *feasibility assessment* is the process of evaluating the possibility of conducting a new research project against the pharmacy CT service's ability to fulfil its requirements.

During those visits, the sponsor or delegate presents the trial protocol, inspects the site facility, equipment, policies, procedures, and other requirements. CT pharmacists must attend and collect the necessary information to determine their capability to support the proposed trial.

Sponsors and CROs may also consider exploring site staffing capacity, as the clinical site's high employee turnover can lead to reduced productivity, increased costs, fractured relationships, and fragile teams.

Examples of feasibility questions for a site personnel resource assessment:

- **How many CTs is a PI conducting at the time of the feasibility visit?** PIs undertaking more than three trials, on top of their clinical work, are unrealistic about the supporting the department's limitless abilities to take on additional responsibilities to facilitate extra projects. For example, a PI overseeing five to seven trials concurrently may not have time to check and approve the pharmacy created trial-specific prescription, thus shifting responsibility to a pharmacist.
- **Is a PI showing a silo mentality?** If yes, trials conduct may and frequently do suffer because operating in a silo and disregarding the supporting departments prior commitments, staffing issues, or a lack of resources does not encourage cooperation, coordination, or collaboration.
- **How many CTs is a full-time coordinator managing?** If CRCs are overloaded, they will heavily rely on CT pharmacists' support, which festers tension, conflict, and distress amongst the team members.
- **How many active trials is the pharmacy CT service managing? How many regular CT pharmacists and technicians are working in the area?** Pharmacy overcommitment and understaffing can imbalance the service scope from participant-centred towards basic trial management.

- **Is there a rotation of pharmacy staff through the CT service? If yes, would they be available or accessible during monitoring visits for queries or clarifications, if required?** Pharmacist rotation through a CT service creates difficulties with prompt clarifications/corrections of incorrect entries during monitoring visits or audits due to their unavailability, preventing straight off resolution of outstanding tasks/issues.

The answers to these questions may shed some light on interdepartmental relationships, communication, and collaboration. Well-developed site teams are essential for successful and cost-effective trial implementation. Fundamentally, the aim of a site feasibility visit is exactly that, to establish the site can conduct the trial within the budget and the timeline whilst maintaining data integrity and participant safety.

The next logical question is whether a site feasibility visit is a one-way process. The pharmacy trial area is inspected, local standard operational procedures are provided, questions answered—all to satisfy the sponsor's requirements.

A healthier practice would be for sponsors/CROs and CT pharmacists to *exchange necessary information* beneficial for both parties. The site pharmacists must compile sufficient information to make an informed evaluation of the project requirements.

What information do they require before confirming their capability to facilitate and manage the pharmaceutical part of a new trial? The minimum is to review the protocol, IB, and IP handling manual to assess the pharmacy staffing and physical resources/equipment against the trial requirements, which would be a more constructive approach.

LESSONS LEARNED:

- The pharmacy CT service feasibility visit is best performed by using a customised questionnaire for gathering relevant information.
- There are no feasibility questionnaires and tools specific for CT pharmacists.
- Minimum information required for a new trial feasibility assessment:
    - Clinical trial protocol, investigator brochure (IB), and an investigational product handling manual (IPHM)
    - Minimum action is to review the IB and then, if necessary, to request an IP safety data sheet
- Additional practical information required:
    - Number of expected participants to be enrolled at a site level (confirm with PI to eliminate information discrepancies)
    - Participant location (inpatients or outpatients)
    - Number of dispensing visits
    - Trial duration and recruitment
    - Is the trial randomised? How will the patients be allocated to intervention or control groups?
    - Is the CT blinded, open label, or single- or double-blinded?
    - Are unblinding procedures outlined in protocol, or does the pharmacy CT service need to create customised blinding plan?
    - Are there any specific pharmacy equipment or facilities that may be required?
    - Does the IP require aseptic preparation?
    - What size storage is required?
    - Does the IP pose any risks requiring particular handling precautions?

Usually, sponsors focus on finding paediatric trained PIs with established credentials and expertise and a suitable pool of potential participants. Furthermore, institutional support and infrastructure are equally essential for a trial implementation. PIs, delegate IP management to the pharmacy. While delegation is implied to superior-subordinate relationship, physicians' and pharmacists' working relationships are not based on hierarchy. Still, teamwork, communication, and collaboration are driven by the same goal—delivering safe and effective health care. Considering that, sponsors and CROs are encouraged to directly approach site CT pharmacists and focus on building more streamlined and flexible processes.

An institutional practice of multidisciplinary assessments of new clinical trials, considering the individual departments and the total site capability concurrently, is more effective for planning and scaling paediatric research at the site level.

A pre sponsor's feasibility, self-assessment of a site's and a supporting department's physical resources, staffing, equipment, insurance, and indemnity requirements to ensure the new project is suitable can result in better performance due to the sense of belonging for all involved.

Whether on-site or virtual, CT pharmacists' inclusion in the new CT feasibility assessment visits and the decision-making process is an efficient way to start a new trial.

Being able to effectively manage service capacity and say no for valid reasons or genuinely address inability is vital to stay on track with other CT obligations without prompt provision of additional staff reinforcement when needed.

The consequences of failing to assess or respond to service capacity limitations may have a direct negative impact during trial implementation, including:

- Compromised quality performance and protocol compliance
- Failure to adhere to GCP requirements
- Unintentional compromising of IP management and dispensing processes
- Compromising CT service financial management, such as irregular or incomplete billing, and overlooked budgets and trial agreements

Improvements in site practices and culture changes to mitigate possible negative obstacles before and during trial execution are directly aligned with the sponsor's goal to get their trials up, recruit in the fastest possible way, and attain quality management.

Unquestionably, improving site feasibility assessment would be invaluable for better site selection and accelerating trial implementation performance, quality, and cost. Post feasibility assessment of the exchanged information, the site is either selected to participate in the trial or rejected. If successful, the next step is the preparation of the budget and the clinical trial agreement (CTA).

CHAPTER SEVEN

Pharmacy Clinical Trial Budget

WHO MANAGES THEM?

'In business, you don't get what you deserve, you get what you negotiate'.

—DR. CHESTER KARRASS

Research tells us that site contract and budget negotiations are the most problematic steps of a site trial start up. It is recognised as a problem area in need of improvements as it accounts for up to 40 per cent of trial commencement delays.[23]

How to improve site contracts and budget negotiation efficiency is beyond the scope of this book. However, I attempt to outline and define some of the main pharmacy fees for trial-related services to enhance familiarisation with them.

There have been suggestions that using a good template may help set contract negotiations up for success. It may, but only if the template is comprehensive and the negotiations are focused on amounts and not on items. Clinical sites genuinely do not respond very well to Pharma standard templates created by them to suit their needs. In addition, feedback gathered from a limited number of sites may not be sufficient. We cannot overlook the variability of practice and funding models. Also, paediatric clinical sites may not conduct a trial with the same fees as the adult sites.

Sound financial management encourages CT service expansion and patients' volume growth while improving quality services, all aligned with *Evolving the Dinosaur.*

By sharing my first-hand experience with rebuilding a financially stressed self-funded service, operating on direct cost recovery from sponsors or other funding entities, I hope to raise awareness about the importance of the pharmacy CT service's financial management.

A comprehensive review and familiarisation with the trial protocol and pharmacy manual is a starting point for budget preparation.

The next step is identifying components to be included in the budget and calculation of the required funds to conduct the trial based on tasks and time taken to complete them. The goal is to prepare a budget, which covers the operational costs of the pharmaceutical part.

The pharmacy fees are determined prospectively, negotiated, agreed upon, and included in the clinical trial agreement (CTA).

Often sponsors forward an offer for pharmacy services. Almost always, the discrepancy between offered and required funds is substantial.

Such discrepancy can be due to:

- Lack of understanding of the fee calculations related to trial-specific tasks and limited insights on the pharmacy services and charges.
- A general presumption that a pharmacy does not charge for IP dispensing; thus, offered fees are for administrative duties and storage only.
- Misinterpretation of the correlation between tasks' requirements, time consumed to fulfil these tasks, and the hourly rate of health professionals performing them.
- A sponsor proposed budget listing only a few or no pharmacy fees is more time- and effort-consuming to finalise due to the apparent unfamiliarity with the charges and their calculation intricacies.

Occasionally, no pharmacy fees on the site proposal can indicate the sponsor's financial difficulties. If CROs manage the project's financials, they may not be fair-minded with site fees. In practice, the more significant the gap between trial requirements and the sponsor/CRO proposed budget, the greater the difficulties to reach an agreement.

Budget negotiation often resembles competitive bargaining, where one party's gain is perceived as the other party's loss. Sponsors/CROs and pharmacists appear to be competing to get the biggest piece from a fixed pie. Both parties' arguments are equally disquieting. A lack of complete understanding of protocol requirements and calculations of time/task and cost/unit time spent on different tasks can lead to high volume of emails exchanges without moving forward.

Pharmacists are not professionally trained in negotiation, but any knowledge can be acquired and practised. On one of my first negotiations, I hit rock bottom after the second email on a Friday afternoon. I spent my weekend learning negotiations tactics, but the more I read, the more my confidence was slipping away. Finally, on Monday morning I rang the other party to explain why we could not accept their proposal. The conversation started with a small talk and finished with my budget finalised. My first lesson was to build trust by showing the person on the other side of the budget negotiation that they are my future partner, and we will work together, not against each other.

Next, I explore the pharmacy fees and what is required to prepare a budget.

THE PHARMACY FEES

Why do we need to include all trial-specific fees for pharmacy services in the budget? Because if something is not in the CTA, sponsors are not obligated to pay for it.

For simplicity, I will break down the pharmacy budget into individual items and discuss each one of them.

SET UP FEE

The set up fee, also known as fixed or upfront cost, is usually invoiced following the site initiation visit. It covers the administrative procedures and tasks performed by CT pharmacists before the trial commences. Therefore, this fee incurs independently from a participant's enrolment.

Main tasks that can be considered in calculating it include but are not limited to:

- CT pharmacist's time for participation in external and internal feasibility meetings
- Participation at site initiation visit
- Time consumed for organising and signing off any pharmacy trial-specific authorisations
- Creation of dispensing summary and customised prescription
- Education of other pharmacy staff
- Completion of IRTs, GCP, or other required training
- Development of trial-specific SOPs, pharmacy budget, and assessments for scientific or ethical approvals, if appropriate

The set up fee is payable when a sponsor withdraws a CT before the agreed start date.

ANNUAL ADMINISTRATIVE FEE (AAF)

The AAF is payable immediately after trial commencement and then yearly, at each anniversary. The start date may be traced by either the date of IP arrival or the SIV date, whichever comes first. The fee is not payable if the trial is open but will not start recruitment immediately. That is the case with clinical trials for very rare paediatric diseases.

Frequently, sponsors/CROs presume a set up fee is used instead of AAF for year one. Regrettably, the two fees are allocated for different sets of tasks. AAF covers the operating expenses associated with the ongoing trial administration, such as organising IP entries into a hospital pharmacy product list or equivalent; setting up IP inventory management on pharmacy-dispensing software to meet trial, hospital, and local legal requirements; IP handling; and managing IP procurement logistics, as required. Other tasks include ongoing liaising with PIs and CRCs; preparing for monitoring visits; performing expiry date checking; quarantining IPs, as per IRT/sponsor notifications; additional training of pharmacy staff, if required during the trial conduct (e.g., protocol amendments, changes to procedures and documentation); and any other trial-related duties which may arise.

When calculating AAF, consideration should be given to the number of anticipated patients to be enrolled. For example, an annual fee for a trial with an anticipated one to two participants would consume less pharmacist time than a trial with hundreds of participants.

REFRIGERATED STORAGE OF IPS

It is an annual fee charged for space, fridges' maintenance, and equipment calibration. Reliable 24/7 temperature monitoring systems are used to ensure IP cold chain requirements are not compromised.

AMBIENT SHELF STORAGE

It is an annual fee charged for space. Temperature monitoring systems are used to ensure IPs are kept in a 24/7 ambient temperature-monitored pharmacy CT room/area.

Daily, weekly, or monthly temperature downloading of the recorded data is required. For convenience, I kept the downloaded data/graphs in a central folder, together with the calibration and annual maintenance certificates.

The temperature monitoring recordings must be up-to-date and available upon request for verification by monitors/auditors. Temperature excursion management and notifications to sponsors are intentionally omitted as forms with instructions, including when and how to quarantine affected IPs, are usually provided in the pharmacy folders. For example, when a temperature deviation from the approved storage conditions was recorded, what worked best for me to obtain prompt IP clearance, was to provide a detailed description of the event, the identified causes, supporting data for the exposure duration, and a brief report of the preventative *measures to avoid future incidents.*

DISPENSING FEES

Dispensing fees are subject to local practice. Sponsors prefer to pay per participant's visit, but it may not be the best option for the CT pharmacy.

When considering suitable options for cost recovery, it is best to keep dispensing charges aligned with the standard institutional dispensing units. My advice is to use justifiable calculations. Generally, a budget prepared in a competent, reasonable, and practical manner is accepted by sponsors/CROs.

I stayed away from incorporating pharmacy dispensing fees into participant's visit payments because per visit fees are paid directly to PIs, requiring internal electronic financial transfers. We team up and collaborate with PIs during trial execution. Internal financial transactions are time-consuming and misaligned with professional relationship building. A humble solution is all pharmacy fees, including dispensing, to be listed in the institutional CTA.

RELABELLING FEE

The relabelling fee is a dollar amount per hour per staff member. It is charged only upon a written sponsor's request if required.

Expiry date updates are common, as IP stability profiles are often developing alongside the trial implementation. IP relabelling may be required for other reasons, too.

SHELF STORAGE OF RETURNS

Shelf storage of returns is an annual fee. Charged for storage of IPs returned by participants, expired, or unfit for use, kept in the CT pharmacy until reconciled by CRAs and either returned to the sponsor or destroyed locally.

PHARMACY ARCHIVING FEE

The pharmacy archiving fee is a one-off fee after the trial closeout for storage of pharmacy records, as per local SOP. The fee is a dollar amount per year for fifteen years, or until the youngest participant turns twenty-five years of age, whichever is longer, for Australia, or as per country/state statute of limitations.

CT CLOSEOUT FEE

The closeout fee is a one-off fee charged at the end of the trial. It covers a CT pharmacist's time consumed on signing off IP accountability logs, organising unused IPs to be returned to the sponsor or be locally destroyed, and arranging the pharmacy records for archiving.

IP DESTRUCTION FEE

The IP destruction fee covers pharmacy staff members' time spent on safe onsite destruction of IPs returned by participants, expired, or otherwise unfit for use. It is calculated as a dollar amount per hour per staff member. A sponsor's written authorisation at the start of the trial is required.

REMOTE MONITORING FEE

The remote monitoring fee is applied for CRAs requests to verify trial documents out of regular on-/off-site monitoring visits. The fee is a dollar amount per hour. An example is a request to scan and email trial accountability logs, the IP balance, and temperature-monitoring recordings between scheduled monitoring visits.

FEE FOR PROCUREMENT OF COMMERCIALLY AVAILABLE MEDICINES

This fee is charged for purchasing commercially available medicines used as a comparator or standard therapy. The charge can be calculated as a price per invoice at the time of purchase, plus a 20 per cent or more handling fee. The invoices are submitted to the sponsor for reimbursement or as agreed.

OTHER FEES

Other fees include a CT pharmacist's time for preparation and packing, if IPs are couriered to participants, or other sites regularly throughout the trial duration. A fixed amount of dollars per occasion, but only when or if required.

Note: sponsors must approve in writing the IP transfer to other sites or return to depot.

A fee for consumables may also be considered if a CT service purchases plastic Ziplock bags, cooler boxes, and medicine administration devices specifically for trial participants' use. One frequently asked question is about the difference between the fee for consumable items and the annual administration fee. They are calculated differently. Consumables are physical items by price, while thc annual admin fee is calculated based on a CT pharmacist's time spent on trial tasks multiplied by an hourly rate.

Indirect cost recovery charges may be applied for CT pharmacists' time spent on administrative tasks. Usually calculated as a dollar amount per hour per staff member of fully absorbed hourly rates. I have not charged them separately but added them to the AAF.

THE PHARMACY BUDGET FOR A NEW CLINICAL TRIAL

Creating a customised budget for pharmacy trial-related services is time-consuming and requires significant attention to detail. Therefore, we must consider the local realities and the study's complexity to calculate our time and effort and balance it with being flexible and competitive.

How to achieve it? We can start with getting familiar with the protocol and other sponsor-provided information.

The next step is to identify items purchased by the pharmacy and tasks that pharmacists will perform throughout the trial.

The information provided in protocols or pharmacy manuals may be incomplete or sometimes conflicting; thus, if additional information or clarifications are required, ask for them. In addition, specific tasks may not be documented or are unknown at the time of budget negotiations.

During budget negotiation, things may not be black and white.

ASSESSMENT OF RESPONSIBILITIES

While we generally know what we do during trial execution, we may not recognise what each new trial's actual expectations and responsibilities are. To obtain additional information and fill in existing gaps, I used a budget questionnaire.

My questionnaire has always been a living document. I regularly added new relevant questions and removed the inapplicable ones, tailoring them to suit each individual trial as needed. My practical advice is to avoid asking questions that have been answered during a feasibility visit, or the answers can be found in the already provided resources. It erodes credibility.

Asking sponsors or their delegates to complete the questionnaire before a feasibility assessment worked much better for preliminary information gathering. I used three types of questions to obtain general information, for budget purposes and inquiries for future service planning. For example, enquiring whether the sponsor is considering an extension of the core trial.

Completed questionnaires are best kept together with finalised CTAs for future reference. If during trial implementation, the service is requested to perform activities that were answered as not required during budget negotiation, they need to be addressed with the sponsor.

Once all necessary information is compiled, we can identify CT pharmacy tasks, estimate the time for performing them, and multiply them by the pharmacist's hourly rates.

To be efficient and effective, we need to be pragmatic. Managing a busy service can be daunting, but it is realistic to continuously improve and scale a service while *Evolving the Dinosaur* and enjoying the results. Indeed, I hope that it would work for others as well as it worked for me.

PHARMACY CUSTOMISED QUESTIONNAIRE

Customised budget questionnaires requires an upfront investment of time and effort. However, preparing an accurate budget ensures appropriate financial support, serves as a road map for invoicing and encourages staff fulfilment and improved performance.

I have included a budget questionnaire example in the appendix, which I have used successfully for years.

It takes time for new sponsors to get familiar with the site pharmacy trial management style and effectiveness or lack thereof. However, my personal experience is that once a CT service has exhibited outstanding management, cost savings, and customer satisfaction, future negotiations with repeated sponsors become relatively straightforward due to established creditability and rapport.

A lack of transparency can lead to a loss of trust. CT/research pharmacists know what they do, why and how long it will take, but the people at the other side of the negotiation may not. Thus, open and sincere communication during budget negotiations is essential.

LESSONS LEARNED:

- The person at the other side of a budget negotiation is a future partner to work with, not against.
- Effective negotiation is a collaborative effort.
- Establish a connection for achieving optimal outcomes for both parties.
- Do all you can to show that you are negotiating in good faith.
- Build trust-based influence, rapport, and mutual understanding.
- Sharpen your conflict resolution skills and have strategies ready if the negotiation does not go as expected.

A few years ago, I negotiated the pharmacy fees for a seasonal clinical trial with a sponsor's budgeting specialist based overseas. It did not take long to understand that we were going in circles over one hundred dollars and away from reaching common ground. Finally, we reached an agreement, but we missed the season, and the trial closed out without enrolling a single participant.

Many other similar experiences over the years have made me wonder how pharmacy budgets could be done more expediently. For example, what do we do when budget negotiation is stalled or the sponsor rejects our proposed fees, despite all efforts?

Ongoing acceptance of unreasonably low pharmacy fees is threatening CT service sustainability and scalability. There is a positive correlation between a trial's complexity and the time consumed for budget negotiation. Sometimes negotiations could go overboard, dragging on and on until hitting a total jam. So, what do we do next? Politely say no because of the unrealistically low fees, or accept them?

When budget negotiation gets jammed, a request for escalation is the way forward in reaching an agreement. However, depending on the clinical trial timelines, some disagreements may require an early mediation to speed up the process before it is too late. Often, PIs' support and request for pharmacy budget finalisation are sufficient for reaching a resolution.

What can we do to avoid lengthy and time-consuming negotiations?

Many pharmacy CT services use predetermined pharmacy fees.

The benefits of using fixed costs are:

- They are available for prompt provision upon request.
- They are perceived as accurate and justified because they have been provided and accepted unchallenged numerous times.
- Pharmacists do not need to read the new trial protocols and seek additional information to perform an immediate assessment of the project requirements.

The main disadvantage is:

- Fixed fees can lead to underbudgeting (the need for high quality research drives up a trial's complexity).

Some of the issues with the current pharmacy fees are:

- The number of fees in a budget affect negotiation length because each individual cost needs approval.
- Raising invoices is time-consuming and an error-prone process. It is impractical to deal with too many fees.
- Electronic billing has its distinctive set of problems. Any omitted fees will not be paid before they are entered into the system.

The answer to the question, *Are CT pharmacists the best people to prepare the pharmacy budgets?* is yes and no! Some pharmacy CT services have attempted to resolve the burden of pharmacy budgeting, negotiating, and billing by delegating the financials to the institutional research centres. It appears to be a convenient option until it is not. Any modification of a fee or wording in the CTA can easily be overlooked by a research person and financially disadvantaged pharmacy fund. A better option is to simplify the budget.

CAN PHARMACY BUDGETS BE SIMPLIFIED AND STANDARDISED?

They can be simplified and still achieve cost recovery. For example, all yearly charges can be combined into a single payment (annual administration fee, IP storage, storage of returns, and consumables). In addition, cost recovery items can be bundled together and charged as a single category every X month(s) or as suitable. Dispensing fees are better reimbursed directly to a pharmacy CT service. What best worked for me was calculating the dispensing costs on both, the time taken for a CT technician to distribute IPs via the pharmacy dispensing system and complete the IPALs, and the time taken for a pharmacist to double-check/sign as per routine practice. And finally, the 'if required fees' (IP destruction, re-labelling, remote monitoring visits, and packaging/organising IP returns to the sponsor) are charged when a service is provided.

The main advantage of a simplified pharmacy budget is time and effort saved for everyone involved, which can be redirected towards more pressing trial matters.

Inter-institutional standardisation is challenging due to variability in hospital practices, policies, and procedures. However, it is not impossible, but it will require a strong collaboration, cooperation, and inclusion of multi-stakeholders.

LESSONS LEARNED:

- Expect sponsors/CROs to question and negotiate each pharmacy fee.
- Be diligent in setting accurate charges and document costs calculations to validate budget queries if required.
- Request realistic and justifiable fees.
- Resist making unreasonable fee reductions.
- Avoid under budgeting. It leads to fund deficit regardless of participants recruitment.
- Verify the pharmacy fees are correct as negotiated before the CTA is executed.
- Establish a billing or electronic funds transfer process during trial set-up as required.
- Cost recovery of pharmacy trial-related services is essential for their ability to continue facilitating a larger volume of more complex paediatric research.

Once the sponsor/CRO accepts, approves, and includes the

pharmacy budget in the CTA, then we can focus on the next step—pharmacy CT set up. Why this stage is essential for the pharmacists is outlined in the next chapter.

CHAPTER EIGHT

New Clinical Trial Set Up

FOR PHARMACISTS BY PHARMACISTS

'We are what we repeatedly do. Excellence, then, is not an act, but a habit'.

—ARISTOTLE

Do your best each day and enjoy the process until it becomes a habit.

This chapter introduces and elaborates on the internal CT pharmacy set up for a new paediatric trial. This multistep process is not standardised and is widely different between hospitals and countries. Over the years, I have been asked repeatedly by sponsors/CRO representatives, 'What does it involve and why are pharmacists engaging in extra work?' So, I hope to provide some insightful information about its purpose and benefits.

So, what is performed during the pharmacy new trial set up?

- Authoring a trial-specific summary/guideline and IP dispensing procedures

- Creating a trial customised prescription (Rx)
- CT pharmacists complete online or face to face training, as required
- Introducing the new trial to. other pharmacy staff and train them
- Developing trial-specific SOPs, if required
- Preparing report/comments or feedback on the trial pharmaceuticals to the EC/IRB, as required

As a non-standardised process, the above list of tasks is not all-inclusive.

The new trial set up is intended to guarantee that essential guides and safeguards are in place for the seamless provision of pharmacy services during trial execution, even if key pharmacy personnel is away. Understandably, external stakeholders may wonder why the pharmacists need to create summaries when sponsors/CROs provide them with pharmacy manuals. A detailed examination of the completeness and quality of information resources provided to pharmacists is outlined in Chapter 9. Meanwhile, I will move straight to what is involved and to how to create a trial or dispensing summary and prescription.

CLINICAL TRIAL CUSTOMISED SUMMARY

A CT pharmacist-created trial summary is intended to serve as a quick reference. Its groundwork includes an extensive review of relevant protocol parts, pharmacy manual, site initiation visit presentation slides, and the investigator's brochure to extract *essential information.*

I am adverse towards the use of trial summaries for several reasons:

- It is an unsafe practice to rely on a summary that may or may not include/contain *all* crucial information.
- It is unsafe to use a summary that may not be updated promptly after each protocol or pharmacy manual amendment, especially when IP doses, frequencies, or other critical information has changed.
- Understaffing, work overload, and time constraints may negatively affect their intended benefits

Before creating a trial summary, we should ask ourselves a few questions: Do we require one in the first place? Who is responsible for the ongoing version control and updates?

One additional question and answer, targeted exclusively at sponsors and CROs, is: Why would CT/research pharmacists create such summaries? The answer is because the IP handling manuals are not precise or do not contain the information, CT pharmacists require to fulfil trial management more confidently.

Currently, site pharmacists do not have a comprehensive one-stop reference.

A practical solution is developing a single trial information resource, exclusively created to satisfy pharmacists' needs, with their input and feedback.

The trial summaries can become outdated and unreliable information resources if no one is in charge. Safe practice can be maintained by establishing a version control system and a dedicated CT pharmacist responsible for timely updates when required. All EC/IRB approved protocol amendments must be forwarded promptly to the pharmacy CT service.

Drafting a new trial's summary before the SIV works better because it allows us to pick out missing or incorrect information/instructions during the initiation visit and make necessary corrections well before trial commencement. In practice, any information or instruction discrepancies between sponsor-provided information resources must be clarified and corrected before enrolling the first participant.

While the practice of creating CT summaries differs between hospital pharmacies, the critical information included in them does not. I have provided a customisable template as an example for readers to compare practice, adopt parts, or copy the entire structure.

CT summaries or dispensing guides must be updated, as required, and version control maintained.

> Note: the comprehensiveness of a trial summary can vary, depending on the service's needs. Monitoring visit frequency and much more can be included. But often, creating a dispensing guide and outlining the local IP dispensing procedure may be sufficient.

The next set up item is to create a trial-specific prescription.

CLINICAL TRIAL-CUSTOMISED PRESCRIPTION

Investigational products are subject to the same local legislation, hospital policies, and procedures as registered medicines. Therefore, IPs cannot be dispensed without a physician's written prescription (Rx) or electronic order.

Creating a trial customised Rx has multiple benefits, such as:

- Offers a clear representation of the clinical visits dispensing visually
- Saves PIs time—if it contains all essential information and is straightforward—can be completed by ticking pre-filled participant visit number and requires minimal additional writing
- More efficient IPs prescribing, dispensing, and checking
- More effective for dispensing billing/funds recovery
- Reduced likelihood of prescribing errors, resulting in increased participant safety

Creating correct, comprehensive, and easy to use prescription is a time-consuming task but is well justified. The best practice is to start the first prescription draft while reviewing the trial materials for budget preparation. Pinning down the number of dispensing visits, frequency, and IP quantity per visit helps calculate costs for the budget and create an accurate Rx.

Customised prescriptions offer a more efficient IP management pathway cycle, averting ordering, prescribing, and dispensing errors, contributing significantly towards *Evolving the Dinosaur*.

LESSONS LEARNED:

- CT prescriptions must be created using the latest approved protocol version, IP handling manual, and other relevant information provided by sponsors/CROs.
- If a computerised provider order entry is used, ensure IP orders are set up and available on the system before the first participant enrolment is due.
- Simplify trial prescriptions as much as practical while keeping all required information, as per protocol.

- Trial Rx must be simple, easy to use and check, and comply with legislative and protocol requirements.
- Each Rx must be double-checked, approved, and signed off by the PI.
- Correct Rx increases participants' accurate and safe use of IPs.

DOSE DISCREPANCIES

Incorrect dose(s) on prescriptions or dose difference(s) between IRT's IP assignment and the Rx must be clarified and corrected. A practical tip is to investigate where the discrepancy may be coming from before contacting the physician.

Do not assume the IRT-assigned dose is always correct. Participant details and other data are entered on a system by a research team member, who may err. Check the previous visit's dosing, body weight, and if the current visit requires a dose adjustment.

Incorrect body weight (BW) leads to wrong doses on Rx or IRT assignment or both. When dose inconsistency is detected, CT pharmacists should not take on the responsibility of deciding which one is correct. Participants' continuous supply with IPs cannot be compromised, but neither can their safety. Indeed, IPs are subject to the same local legislation, hospital policies, and procedures for safe prescribing and dispensing as registered medicines.

I have included a trial Rx template for visual illustration in the appendix, but it can be modified, individualised, and used for other IP forms.

TRIAL SPECIFIC TRAINING FOR PHARMACISTS

During the new CT set up, CT pharmacists complete various online or face to face training to disseminate knowledge, educate, and train other pharmacy staff and health professionals on the investigational product administration, safety, and handling precautions. Specific administrative duties may be assigned internally to pharmacy technicians, but the lead/senior CT pharmacist remains responsible for compliance with local laws and regulations for their work. However, the CT pharmacist's educational role across other research or clinical staff is yet to be established and standardised at a site level, much less universally.

Often, sponsors require pharmacy specific standard operational procedures (SOPs). Thus, I offer a step-by-step process of how to create them. Unfortunately, inter-institutional variety, in practice, does not support standardisation.

PHARMACY CLINICAL TRIAL SERVICE—SPECIFIC SOPS

SOPs are detailed and specific written instructions describing how routinely performed operations are completed—who does what, when, why, where, and how. They serve to document what has been adopted as standard practice.

The most frequently requested SOPs I have been asked to provide are IP temperature monitoring, IP destruction, IP blinding, and archiving of pharmacy documentation. Additionally, SOPs for transferring IPs from X to Y, dispensing, and re-labelling, are desirable. Finally, for hospital accreditation purposes, a complete set of service SOPs may be required.

How do we create them? The included SOP structure is practice-tested and has been accepted by sponsors over many years.

- Introduction, objectives, and purpose
- Glossary and acronyms
- Scope
- Ownership and responsibility, for example:
    - 'Applies to all clinical research personnel involved in....'
    - 'Personnel responsible for...when delegated by PI'
- Background
- Procedure: how it is done
- Dissemination and implementation
- Monitoring compliance and effectiveness
- Review and updating—for example, 'This SOP will be reviewed every X year, or whenever there are changes to legislation or working practices that impact the content.'

Also, there may be other conditions specifying the possibility of an SOP to be merged with another, if appropriate, or removed, if it becomes redundant. The key points are that SOPs must describe how trial-related activities are performed from start to end and precisely state where, who does what, when, why, and how.

Significant virtual solutions have advanced during and post COVID-19, which may necessitate the site's pharmacy services to focus on SOPs related to remote work SOPs, ensuring trial participants' safety and compliance are maintained. Shifting to virtual clinical trials certainly adds new challenges for paediatric research.

CHAPTER NINE

Pharmacy Clinical Trial Folder

INFORMATION RESOURCES

'What the world needs to understand is the inverse relationship between productivity and paperwork. Unquestionably, COVID-19 brought to light that paper-based trials and manual processes are not sustainable for the future'.

—VIOLET FORD

This chapter attempts to address the imposed challenges on site pharmacists by the information resources created and provided by sponsors/CROs. By surveying the problems and suggesting some solutions, I hope readers gain insight into the work and the pain points of CT pharmacists with whom they may be less familiar. The topic of what the content of a pharmacy manual should be to support adult clinical trial protocols is not new and has been well known. However, that is not the case with paediatric trials, and improvements are yet to be seen.

I intentionally omit commentary on the entire contents of the pharmacy folder, as they are reasonably standard, but instead I focus on the suitability of pharmacy IP handling manuals and the issues surrounding the investigational product accountability logs (IPALs).

Are they created for the intended users?

THE PHARMACIST PLAYBOOK

'The way we do anything, is the way we do everything'.

—MARTHA BECK

Investigational product handling manual (IPHM) or pharmacy manual is a booklet of IP handling and management instructions intended to be a hands-on reference. It is supposed to be the CT pharmacist's bible.

So let us canvass its contents and go through possible solutions to eliminate the need for pharmacist-created trial summaries.

Pharmacy manuals are not a one-stop information resource. They are intended for pharmacists but are actually created by external stakeholders without the user's input or feedback. Their present status of being an unreliable or incomplete source of information is a significant pain point. The lack of pharmacist-specific information all in one place is counterproductive when time-sensitive information retrieval is desired. Also, it can affect CT service metrics. For example: if time spent per enquiry is measured, incomplete and missing information or discrepancies between pharmacy manual, protocol, or other sources influence the assessment accuracy. In the absence of built-in feedback loops between CT pharmacists and sponsors/CROs, incorrect information or errors are reported locally, but it is unclear if and how, or by whom, they are assessed or taken on board for future improvements.

A practical corrective step is to transform the pharmacy manuals into a customised *one-stop information resource.* However, before looking at improvements, it is essential to address the identified pitfalls.

Often, it appears the pharmacy manuals are either created too early when not all essential information is available or in a hurry at the last minute by individuals who are not versed with what is necessary for the primary users—the CT pharmacists.

What is the worst scenario I have ever seen? The protocol points to the IP handling manual for detailed information, but the information is neither detailed nor complete.

What should a pharmacy manual be? A precise and practical hands-on reference for the intended users who require accurate and concise information and instructions of up to a point—what, when, how, and why. If that is achieved, pharmacist created summaries may not be required. The immediate benefits are that sponsors/CROs are reducing the pharmacy set up fee and freeing up pharmacists' time for other activities.

Let us look at an example of information routinely provided in pharmacy manuals: 'The interactive response technology (IRT) will be used for study drug receipt confirmation, inventory management, study drug subject assignments, dispensing, screening/screen failure tracking, and emergency unblinding'.

A CT pharmacist needs to know only the actions they are performing. For some trials, the pharmacists may only receive IPs and see what is assigned to participants. In many instances, the pharmacists are not even granted access to generate a site IP inventory report. This was a case when a scheduled one-hour audit visit dragged on over half a day because the auditor requested a site IP inventory report, but no one from the team had access to this particular IRT function. Indeed, no one could explain why pharmacists did not have access to generate an inventory report. The CRA was the only person with access.

General descriptions and instructions, such as 'Study drug subject assignments, dispensing…', are better avoided, as they lead to questions, such as: 'What is the difference between the two actions and who does what?' Pharmacists do not always assign investigational products to participants on IRTs, and the assigned IPs are not dispensed via IRTs but by a pharmacy dispensing software. Thus, indicating who does what would dispel ambiguity.

RELEVANT INFORMATION

Pragmatic improvements through content management can transform pharmacy manuals to serve as the only comprehensive information resource to guide CT pharmacists throughout trial execution.

What relevant information should be included:

- Contact details of sponsor/CRO
- Clinical Trial synopsis
- Investigational Product Details
- Name
- Form: tablets, solution, suspension, vials, etc., including description of the formulation and excipients
- Strength(s)

- Packaging box/bottle (X tablets): box of X injections, blister, bottle 250 mL, etc.
- Size of the packaging (for storage considerations and solutions)
- IP labels samples, including for reconstituted products

IP ADMINISTRATION INSTRUCTIONS

What essential information should a customised pharmacy manual contain?

Special instructions for injectable IPs requiring reconstitution, dilution, or aseptic manufacturing:

- The details of diluents, for example, water for injection (WFI) or 0.9 per cent sodium chloride or another specific diluent.
- The container's type and size, an infusion bag, size (50 mL or 100 mL), and the final infusion concentration. For paediatric patients, specifying *maximum concentration or minimum volume* is essential.
- IP's compatibility with other medicines and/or infusion equipment, if applicable.
- Requirement to use filters, giving sets, infusion bags, etc., and their specifications. Who provides them? The sponsor or purchased locally?
- Information about any particular precautions to be taken during reconstitution/dilution or (aseptic) preparation (i.e., use of filters and protection from light).
- The maximum dose, route, and rate of administration, as applicable.
- Storage conditions and precautions post reconstitution/dilution.

- Information about the *management of extravasation injuries*, if available.
- Participant monitoring requirements post IP administration and duration. Who can perform it? Is the PI required to be physically present during the observation period?
- Information about an unopened product and shelf life post reconstitution, dilution, etc.
- Clear instructions about discarding used or partially used vials of monoclonal antibodies and other hazardous IPs. These must not be kept at the site pharmacy for accountability per occupational health and safety regulations.

Note: if outer boxes are sufficient for IP reconciliation, well-defined directions effectively increase CT pharmacist confidence to appropriately discard used or partially used products without doubts about compromising IP accountability.

Special instructions and information for oral IPs:

- The number of liquid oral IP bottles assigned via IRT and dispensed depends on the daily dose, IP concentration, bottle size, and supply duration. The use of standardised dosing milligram/microgram/BW/*dose* is safer than milligram/microgram/BW/*day* in divided doses.
- Specify if IP dispensing is per IRT assignment to eliminate discrepancies between prescriptions and IRT assignments due to calculation differences and volume rounding.
- Consider providing emergency or backup supply to compensate for bottle spillage or breakage and outline when IPs are dispensed and quantity.
- Provide clear and precise administration directions and any special instructions, for example, with fatty food.
- Provide information on *IP's interactions with milk.*

- List or table all known food, herbal, or other interactions for a quick reference and prompt information retrieval.
- List or a table of all known IP interactions with other medications.
- Advice about the best action post-missed and vomited doses.
- Advice about post-management of first dose *allergic/hypersensitivity reactions.*
- Information about known IP side effects requiring rescue treatment with other medicines. For example, IP reduces calcium and vitamin D levels, necessitating supplementation.

CT pharmacists must be aware of vaccines, special tests, and rescue treatments required to budget for them than engage in budget re-negotiation during the implementation. Frequently, such inconveniences are shared by all affected parties—PIs, CT pharmacists, participants, monitors, and sponsors.

INSTRUCTIONS TO COMPLETE IP ACCOUNTABILITY LOGS

Accountability logs, paper or electronic, should be free of ambiguous instructions or functionality, causing unnecessary confusion. Electronic processing of IP returns should be empowering clinical site teams; however, if no one understands what quantity to enter because the system is irresponsive, the intended improved data collection is lost. For example, an IRT respond on inputting one box, but the IPs are boxes of ninety sachets, and the participants returns range from one to ninety per box; we have a tech-related issue, enforcing counter productiveness and substandard data collection due to the poorly designed electronic logs and a lack of clear instructions. CRAs may not offer prompt advice or even understand what the issue is, resulting in further inconveniences and delays in completing accountability and participant IP compliance.

Other similar examples:

- Instructions to stick cut off parts of IP container's labels on logs and provide logs without spaces for those cut off parts.
- Or providing logs with spaces for cut off labels for IP containers without cut off portions on labels.

INSTRUCTIONS FOR IP STORAGE

- Storage during transportation from site to participant's homes: Is the sponsor providing carry bags, cooler bags, or boxes?
- Storage during transportation from CT pharmacy to clinical sites: Are there specific precautions or a chain of custody requirement?
- Advise if IP temperature monitoring recording is performed per sponsor's instructions or per site temperature monitoring SOP.
- Outline the action plan and provide forms for temperature excursion management and reporting.
- Specify if affected IPs require both physical and IRT quarantining. Standardised information for international, multisite studies is essential.

INSTRUCTIONS ABOUT MISSING OR LOST IPS

Provide instructions and clearly outlined steps or a process to be followed to manage missing or unintentionally lost IPs. CT pharmacists are usually the first point of contact about IP related queries by parents/caregivers, CRCs, PIs, and other health professionals.

IP SPILL MANAGEMENT PROCESS

It has been noted that very few pharmacy manuals contain information about the management of IP spillages on surfaces, clinical personnel, patients, or parents and caregivers, even if there are no specific safety issues. Concerns about IP contamination is frequently questioned internally by different stakeholders. Thus, I attempt to raise this point. Practical and rapidly accessible information about IP spill management is essential, because not finding information does not guarantee safety.

INFORMATION ABOUT ADVERSE DRUG REACTIONS (ADRS)

A list or table of the most common ADRs or a reference to the relevant IB pages for quick information retrieval would be sensible. When a trial participant is hospitalised, the institutional clinical staff habitually contact pharmacists first about the IP safety profile. To provide prompt information or create an IP safety summary, an up-to-date list of ADRs is fundamental, as gathering it from multiple resources is a slow, time-consuming, and ineffective process but remediable without the need to reinvent the wheel.

IP ORDERING, SHIPMENTS, RECEIPTS, AND RELEASE

- Specify IPs first supply, subsequent ordering, and the items included in the shipment. For example, a Sensitech TempTale 4 (TT4) USB monitor.
- Include applicable instructions such as:
    - Immediately upon receipt, stop the temperature monitoring device.
    - Verify container/kit numbers and check them against the shipping invoice/packing slip.

- Register receipt of the shipment via IRT (name).
    - Download the data from temperature monitoring devices.
    - Print a copy of downloaded temperature recording and file with shipping documents.
    - Forward copies to specified parties via email or upload to a cloud storage platform.

Note: not all clinical sites are able to fax documents.

- Stipulate a time frame for IP acknowledgement receipt via the IRT. For example, within four hours or no later than twenty-four hours or within the same working day or as soon as practical!
- Advise if IRT-generated *shipping request* and *shipment receipt* notifications should be filed in the pharmacy folder, for practice consistency.
- Ensure clinical site IRT login flexibility is maintained. IRT generated shipping requests should be forwarded to more than one pharmacist to ensure continuity is sustained when one staff member is away or leaves work. Site team members must be provided with IRT logins to essential functions. Restrictions on how many people can login are impractical and hinder site team's efficiency.

STANDARD THERAPY AND ANCILLARY SUPPLY

- Specify what standard therapy medicines or ancillary supplies would be required and how they would be resupplied: automatically or manually by the sponsor or by the CT pharmacy.
- Provide IPs and ancillary item dimensions for site storage

preparedness. Unanticipated requests for storage of large volumes or bulky supplies may not be accommodated if not replanned.

- Specify the necessity for an individual, participant-specific supplies, which may require different storage solutions in the pharmacy to avoid IP mix-ups and errors.
- Specify who provides the ancillary supplies to participants. If pharmacists, indicate the quantities to be handed out and at which visits to avoid omissions and inconveniences to participants and caregivers due to insufficient supplies to cover their needs between visits.

IP DISPOSITION: SITE DESTRUCTION OR RETURN TO SPONSOR/SUPPLIER

Destruction of empty or partially used containers and expired IPs traditionally has been performed by the site pharmacists, post IP accountability and reconciliation. Usually, the CRA would authorise the destruction and sign off the local destruction form(s) along with a CT pharmacist. However, I want to comment on some new initiatives requiring PIs and pharmacists to approve the onsite IP destruction.

While there has not been an official change of practice, the influx of insufficiently trained or inexperienced CRAs has changed the landscape. In addition, persistent unreasonable or peculiar demands can have a negative and demoralising impact on clinical site teams.

A simple and effective solution would be to create guidelines on how IP disposition is handled at the site level and who does what. Standardised practice is best achieved by providing explicit instructions in the trial materials. For example, the CRA performs reconciliation and then authorises the IP disposition form. A CT pharmacy staff member double-checks and signs it.

Standardised information and training are of paramount importance for consistent, efficient, and effective trial management. There should *not* be gaps and discrepancies in operational procedures between the sponsor, CRO/CRA, and site team.

Likewise, if electronic processing of returned, expired, and unfit for use IPs is required, clear instructions must be given. Knowing who is performs what and when dispels confusion, practice variance, and conflicts between site team members and CRAs.

During trial implementation, there should not be discrepancies between instructions and actions. For example, a written direction that a CRA will retrieve original accountability logs from the pharmacy folder during the monitoring visit should be actioned. If not, it creates ambiguities and raises questions about the rationality of instructions and performance.

In conclusion, explicit information, instructions, and well-defined directions should be provided to all parties involved regarding who completes/does what, when, and why.

BLINDED CLINICAL TRIALS AND BLINDING PLAN

Next, I will outline the general pharmacy practice with blinded trials and how CT pharmacists ensure it is maintained. The topic is relatively sensitive for external stakeholders, and I have frequently been asked to create a customised blinding plan. Hopefully, the detailed information will provide clarity and reassurance for the external trial stakeholders, who may be less familiar with general CT pharmacy practice.

The most important questions for the clinical site teams are:

- What are the decoding procedures for an emergency reveal of an investigational product without breaking the blind for the remaining participants' treatment?
- Who can authorise it and unblind a participant?
- Which members of the site team are blinded/unblinded?
- Is there a blinding plan provided by the sponsor, or will a standard pharmacy CT service blinding SOP be used?

For international, multisite trials, a sponsor-provided blinding plan works best for practice standardisation. Otherwise, CT pharmacists create site-specific IP dispensing and handling guidelines, SOP, or a customised blinding plan. Usually, pharmacy staff are unblinded, while other clinical site personnel with direct participant care responsibilities are blinded to treatment assignment; thus they:

- Minimise, as much as possible, direct communication and interactions between blinded and unblinded personnel to avoid accidental revealing of a participant's treatment assignment.
- Ensure that active and placebo IPs are identical in appearance, labelling, preparation time, expiry time/date, dose, dosing interval, and instructions for administration. If required, matching covers for light protection and the same needles and filters for administration are provided.

What roles and responsibilities do the unblinded staff have? What practices can potentially prevent unblinding or identifying treatments?

All research team members are blinded to study treatment

assignments in double blinded CTs until all participants complete treatments and the database is locked.

When CT pharmacists are unblinded, their dispensing procedures ensure that all necessary steps are taken to prevent accidental unblinding.

Below is an example of a dispensing process of an injectable IP for a blinded trial:

- Once the prescription/order is forwarded to the pharmacy, the unblinded pharmacy staff dispense as per IRT assignment and label active and placebo IP doses, syringes, or bags *with the same, unrevealing pharmacy labels: investigational product (name) or placebo (strength) + study name + administration directions + expiry + other required information.*
- The unblinded pharmacist ensures appropriate masking of the IP before releasing it to blinded team members for administration.
- The pharmacy folder and all used IP containers, kits, vials, syringes, or packs are retained in a dedicated place, inaccessible for blinded personnel until an unblinded monitor performs accountability and reconciliation.
- With aseptic manufacturing, the preparation method may be documented on a pharmacy computer-generated manufacturing sheet and only unblinded monitors can review its correctness and the log entries.
- Once dispensing is completed, the IP is placed in appropriate packaging and into a particular hard-shell container, cool icebox, or bag for transportation to the place of use. The blinded CRC must contact the unblinded pharmacist to confirm dispensing is completed and arrange a pickup time from the pharmacy.

- If accidental unblinding occurs, it must be reported immediately, using an accidental unblinding form.

IP STORAGE AND ACCOUNTABILITY IN BLINDED CTS

The general practice is as follows:

- Maintaining secure storage of all active and placebo IPs with limited access.
- Ensuring appropriate receipt, handling, and temperature monitoring.
- Maintaining blinded IP accountability logs, as required.
- Storing IPs, including all used/returned, in a dedicated place that is inaccessible to the blinded personnel
- IP reconciliation is performed by an unblinded monitor.

BLINDED/UNBLINDED PERSONNEL AND FACILITY

- All pharmacists/pharmacy staff involved must be adequately trained and aware of the importance of maintaining trial blindness.
- Limited access to the pharmacy trial records, dispensing, accountability logs, and treatment assignments by blinded personnel is ensured and maintained at all times.
- CT pharmacists ensure the unblinded monitor's email address is only accessible to unblinded staff.
- Restrict access of blinded research team members during unblinded pharmacy monitoring visits.
- PI and other blinded team members must not be copied on correspondence between unblinded CT pharmacists and unblinded CRAs.

INTERACTIVE RESPONSE TECHNOLOGY—PITFALLS AND SOLUTIONS

IRT has empowered sponsors to manage critical aspects of their clinical trials, including enrolment/randomisation, dosing and IP assignments, supplies, IP inventory management, unblinding, and so on. Dosing algorithms allow IP assignments to participants, as per protocols' dosing schedules and treatment arms. A more complex dosing algorithm may be required in paediatric trials due to body weight-based dosing and age consideration.

I want to share a few practice-identified issues with IRTs. Some, if not all of them, can be brought to an end and eliminate the clinical site teams' frustration with the technological solutions intended to empower, not disempower.

DOSE CALCULATIONS AND SAFETY

IRTs for paediatric CTs must have a *feature for dose calculation* and *maximum dose capping* to ensure obese or overweight participants do not receive more than they should. That was the case in a CT with a product registered for adults with a known maximum dose of X mg per week. There was no surprise that the IRT printout suggested an amount higher than the maximum adult dose, as the patient was steadily gaining weight over time. While the participant was dispensed the correct dose, the site team was burdened in correspondence, queries, and paperwork due to dose discrepancy between the electronic assignment and the physician order/pharmacy dispensing.

UNSCHEDULED PARTICIPANT VISITS

Pharmacy manuals should provide information about unscheduled visits and how they are managed to avoid delays in IP supply. For example, when can it happen and what process is followed? Such enquiries are almost always directed to CT pharmacists, but they do not always have the answers.

When it comes to an IRT choice for a new trial, the cost is an essential factor, but so are capability, functionality, and appropriateness for the particular trial. However, it appears that the price is the determining factor. For sure, selecting an IRT that does not provide all the required functionality is less cost-effective in the long run if it does not save time and on IP supply costs. For example, the site's inability to access unscheduled visit function and assign IPs as a backup supply created a mini disaster. The research coordinator and I spent over four hours contacting various external parties to organise an emergency supply. Unfortunately, we did not have access to the system's unscheduled visit feature as it was not paid for and thus not available to us. The result was that the participant waited too long and was inconveniently sent home without IPs. The sponsor paid for the function in question, including for fridge monitored home delivery. Indisputably, the actual cost savings were wiped off.

Participants' unscheduled visits should be considered during new clinical project planning and IRT vendor selection.

INVESTIGATIONAL PRODUCT ACCOUNTABILITY LOGS (IPALS)—ISSUES AND SOLUTIONS

CT pharmacists maintain accurate records of received, dispensed, returned, and disposed of IPs throughout a trial's implementation. All performed transaction details are recorded on the accountability logs. Regular inventory counts are completed for each IP to confirm transactions accuracy, meaning the physical quantity on hand matches the total balance recorded on the IPAL. Any discrepancies are investigated promptly and reported to the sponsor or their delegate.

Accountability logs are provided by sponsors or CROs. But if considered unsuitable, due to lack of columns to document specific transactions, CT pharmacists can create their own. Sponsor approval is required to use site created logs.

Trial customised logs support accurate IP data recording, and when they are not, CT pharmacist's and monitor's productivity and efficiency are negatively impacted. Hopefully, addressing the most problematic and frequent issues will bring about future improvements because if we do not identify, understand, and resolve the existing problems with the paper logs, we cannot create problem-free digital solutions.

One unaddressed question in all pharmacy manuals is whether we should use a new log for each different IP batch/lot number. In case of suspected or actual adverse drug reaction related to a specific IP batch, referring to a single log is the fastest and most convenient way to track and quarantine a product when required.

When dispensing different IP batches, packaging each one separately and counselling patients to use the IP with a closer expiry date first is an effective way of tracking IP use by batch/lot numbers.

Regardless of whether to record different batches on separate logs, specifying it in the pharmacy manual clarifies how the IP logs are completed and eliminate practice discrepancies across sites.

The IPALs are source documents, and as such, if corrections are made, they must be marked with a line through the error entry, then signed and dated. Additional clarifications can be made in the comment column.

While participant accountability logs are self-explanatory, site logs, also known as master logs, often create confusion. It has been noted that occasionally monitors do not understand them, resulting in misinterpretations, never-ending clarifications, and correspondence back forth. In some instances, IPALs management may turn into a total disaster. For example, I have received a request for all site IPALs to be rewritten and back signed five years into a long-term trial, due to log's modifications.

During the SIV, CT pharmacists inspect accountability logs, clarify issues, and provide feedback as required. The impression is that the feedback loop is broken, and changes do not happen quickly enough. Fancy looking logs are often either not suitable for the trial or impractical, or both.

IPALs, whether paper or electronic, should be self-explanatory, neither requiring detailed instructions on how to be completed nor creating confusion between the people completing them and the people verifying them.

CURRENT PROBLEMS:

Lack of 'total balance' column are problematic because they prevent site CT pharmacists from prompt detecting IP balance discrepancies and resolving or reporting them to sponsors.

Inappropriate IPALs. The protocol requires cut-off labels to be stuck on logs, which have either unsuitably sized spaces (too big / too small) or an incorrect number of spaces. For example, to fit ten label cut-offs into logs with four spaces. The opposite scenario is to stick cut-off portions on logs, while the IP labels do not have a cut-off portion. Predictably such situations are managed with unnecessary manual handwriting of IP strengths, kit numbers, lot numbers, and expiry dates. Over decades, it has been established that in healthcare, data transcription leads to human errors. Statistics show that medication transcribing errors are between 11 and 21 per cent. Inappropriate IPALs compel an increased risk of human error during the manual transcribing of six- to eight-digit numbers on several logs, in addition to consuming excessive amounts of time for verification.

Participants' IP returns recording *on master accountability logs* creates reluctance, and no one completes it before the end of the trial. CT pharmacists enter the returned IPs on the participants' logs and the IRT if required.

Is more of the same data better? Is it necessary for returned IPs to be recorded on two sets of logs and then on a destruction form and finally processed electronically on the IRT? What is the end goal of four entries of the same data? I will leave this question open-ended.

Keeping in mind that IPALs record an IP's chain of custody and serves as a tracking document from the time it leaves the sponsor/manufacturer until it is used, destroyed, or returned to the sponsor, so they must be designed to do precisely that. Unsuitable and impractical logs lead to setbacks during trial execution and increased costs. The more unsuitable they are, the more pharmacist and monitor/auditor time is spent on completion and verification.

Various challenges already burden paediatric clinical research. So why not provide clinical sites with IRTs and IPALs that can meet the unique protocol's needs?

LESSONS LEARNED:

- Customised IPALs improve data accuracy, increase monitor/auditor verifications efficiency; thus, is more cost effective.
- Insert N/A instead of having empty spaces on the IPALs.
- Include a participant identification number
- The 'disposition' column on IPALs requires instructions about who completes what. For example, monitor completes 'returned to sponsor' or 'destroyed onsite' on master accountability logs. If not assigned to someone, no one completes it.
- Instructions about who enters expired, damaged, or otherwise unfit for use IPs on IPALs and IRTs is necessary to dispel confusion and assign data entry responsibility to someone.
- IPALs without page numbers (one of X) become messy as the trial advances. It is challenging to arrange them sequentially by following entry dates if not completed manually.
- Shipments recording standardisation on IPALs. What is the best practice? How are shipments recorded? By batch/lot number, expiry date, container number, shipment IDs, or others? If not specified, it is open for individual interpretation and preference, and inter-sites recording variation is inevitable.

IPALs should reflect IP storage requirements, ambient or fridge, and whether they are a blinded or unblinded document. Data entry is performed at the time of occurrence; thus, omitted entries should include both dates—the date of the entry and the date of the event occurrence and a comment that the entry was performed retrospectively.

PART THREE

Tracking

CHAPTER TEN

Ongoing Service Monitoring

HOW TO TRACK PROGRESS

'If you can measure it, you can improve it'.

—PETER DRUCKER

Throughout the first two parts of the book, we explored how to perform a baseline CT service assessment: choose metrics and measure them. Now I will delve into ongoing CT service performance monitoring and tracking.

Although this book is not a theoretical exploration of the monitoring, tracking, or evaluation concepts, I want to present a few basic descriptions. *Monitoring* involves the ongoing measuring of pre-identified performance indicators. It is the process of continuous data collection that provides information on the extent of progress and the success of the implemented improvements. However, it does not tell us if we are getting the right results. *Tracking* is analysing the input and results' data, which allowed me to see exactly how the services and processes performed and how participants/parents/other customers experienced them. In other words, monitoring involved continuous data gathering and tracking to check if the implemented changes were satisfactory and on schedule to meet my goals.

After defining the metrics for base-level and ongoing service performance, performing the ongoing measurements, and logging them in the tracking tool, we can move to the next step of tracking the progress.

Something to keep in mind is that the quality of our original questions must be aligned to the service goals to collect quality answers that will lead to value-added CT service improvements.

Let us delve again into the KPIs, metrics, and measures because they are used as indicators of how the CT service performance was achieved and assessed. Without identifying appropriate key performance indicators, measuring, and then tracking them over time, we would be in the dark about our service performance. It might feel like we are successful, but we will not know by how much and compared to what. We know metrics are trackable, but which ones should we track? Which KPIs can measure the CT service's strategic and operational goals? KPIs measuring strategic objectives inform us where we are now to where we want to be at a certain point in time. The KPIs measuring operational objectives are monitoring our daily operational services delivery. For example, what is a suitable KPI for pharmacy CT service? Is reducing the number of medication errors measurable? Is getting them to zero across all site's active trials a realistic goal?

While data collected through tracking and monitoring inform us if the improvements have been implemented well and whether we are on track to meet our goal, evaluation is focused on demonstrating the impact of improvements. The evaluation confirms if we are doing the right things and is a measure of the service performance. Although different, evaluation complements monitoring. Because it is a more detailed and time-consuming activity, I mainly relied on monitoring to identify potential problems that required attention.

Pharmacy CT service's operational metrics are data points that provide insights on the progress of service performance.

LESSON LEARNED:

The distilled experiences from my journey that lead to practical results are:

- To define the start and endpoint (time frame).
- To clearly define metrics.
- To use effective analytics methods to support achieving targeted improvements.
- To use past performance data to drive the decisions for future improvements.
- To define the measuring unit and measure consistently to allow comparison over time.
- To search for patterns in the data that encourage sound decision making.
- To track operational performance that empowers more targeted decisions boosting service efficiency, effectiveness, and productivity or adjustments as required.
- To determine which metrics to track by continuously keeping in mind which questions we are answering and why, and how the answers will benefit the service.

WHICH KEY METRICS TO TRACK

While a busy pharmacy managed CT service may have many questions to be answered and operational performance metrics, it is best to focus on the meaningful ones and the most beneficial for the service.

I tracked metrics mainly to:

- Identify processes requiring further improvements
- To compare data over time
- Track the progress

I hope this chapter inspires other CT services to adopt and build in tracking metrics over time in their processes, if not already a regular practice, as the benefits outweigh the effort.

I used standard CT pharmacist tasks to illustrate how specific KPIs and metrics can improve certain service processes.

For example, CT pharmacists can use data to drive practice change which shortens pharmacy monitor visit duration. Other suitable metrics to guide the change are the number of errors on logs per monitoring visit and the number of incorrect accountability events of returned IPs, which required corrections.

> Note: tracking data for comparison over a period indicates improvement, decline, or no change.

Tracking CT service performance is valuable not only for service delivery improvements but also for understanding its operations better.

Tracking financial metrics can be used to improve trial budgeting and to assess the service financial capability to fund additional staff.

Tracking the CT pharmacist to participant ratio denotes staff capacity, which directly impacts quality services delivery. For example, if one full-time equivalent (FTE) pharmacist is providing services to many patients, he/she may not be able to deliver safe and high quality services. I have used this metric per day, per month, and year to assess short- and long-term staff requirements.

Tracking communication between CT pharmacists and PIs / clinical research coordinators establishes how frequently site team members communicate with one another. Increased communication enhanced participants' safety and standard of services. It can be measured qualitatively by assessing the team members satisfaction or quantitively by the number of documented communication activities and duration.

Tracking participants' satisfaction was related to my goal to achieve zero wait time for IP dispensing for outpatient clinical visits. Research informs that wait time hurts customer satisfaction. After a long and full-on clinical visit, parents collecting their child's IPs immediately (zero wait time) was associated with high satisfaction, especially when their IP-related questions or concerns were addressed. Assessment of task duration and reasons leading to increased wait time also may need to be considered.

The number of dispensing IP errors is measured by the number of actual errors made by CT pharmacists. Assessment of the error type and reasons leading to it, is essential for corrective and preventative actions. Nil errors also indicate an individual employee's effectiveness and attention to detail, which should also be measured. Feedback, training, coaching, and individual pharmacist KPIs are significant builds that can help improve this metric versus existing performance.

For tracking improvement of participants' safety, I measured the number of *prevented* investigational product errors or risks, which may have led to harm. Data comparison over time reveals improvement, decline, or no change.

Effective tracking of near misses shows the success of current mitigating strategies or the need for review and practice adjustments to drive improvements.

CT service effectiveness was assessed *on the extent* and *time* to which planned improvements were actually achieved.

STAFFING SOLUTIONS BASED ON TIME TRACKING: DOES IT WORK?

An adequate number of appropriately trained paediatric CT pharmacists is critical for successfully managing the pharmaceutical part of clinical trials at sites.

In the absence of international standards and calculation formulas for optimal staffing, I decided to explore if the pharmacy CT services workload could be analysed by tracking time spent on specific trial-related tasks. Then I made a rough estimate of the hours consumed per trial and multiplied it by the number of active trials. It does not sound very encouraging but performing time tracking for one relatively simple trial and one complex was sufficient to obtain reliable figures. Time per task measurements was not done as a project but as part of service change management, mainly for future CT budgeting. Recording those time/task measurements on my tracking tool was a tiny additional job. For example, time for aseptic and non-aseptic manufacturing was obtained straight from the sponsor's forms requiring start and finish time of infusion or dose preparation. Thus, it is not about extensive-time tracking of each activity but sufficient volume and variety to obtain reliable data. If you are already doing it, that is great; otherwise, information on the different methods—manual or using software or apps, including their pros and cons—can easily be found on the internet.

Establishing the maximum number of CTs or the number of participants one FTE CT pharmacist can manage is imperative to avoid an unsafe practice prone to medication errors.

It not only adversely impacts the trial data integrity but also professional standards and employee morale. There are other factors to be considered for appropriate substantiation of a CT service's actual staffing needs. For example, the service scope, whether it provides basic or end-to-end service, including operational and financial management, participation in institutional committees for review and feedback of new CT protocols and participants' IP counselling.

Also, the CT service capacity, which is the volume of research it can handle while maintaining high quality standards and satisfactory performance, needs to be examined thoroughly. Service capacity is not static and changes over time. As an illustration, when I started managing the service, the internal to external sponsored trials ratio was 50:50, which shifted to 30:70 in less than a year. The same PIs moved forward with pharma-sponsored research projects once their internal ones closed out, affecting the service capacity. It increased as local pharmacy IP manufacturing, a time-consuming task, was no longer required. Understanding this upfront helps drive the overall strategic planning of the service.

Complex CTs with aseptic IP preparation require a separate assessment due to the involvement of pharmacy staff from another area with aseptic training and validation. Finally, thought should be given to how paediatric investigational product dose calculations and dispensing must be double-checked independently by two pharmacy staff members.

Keeping all of that in mind, it appears that CT service staffing requirements need more holistic assessment considering the varying nature and changes in the intensity of the workloads.

What would an appropriate number of trials be per one full-time pharmacist? Defining a sensible number of pharmacists to manage service is not a straightforward calculation. My experience is that a quick imbalance of service functionality from average to chaotic or in distress can happen over a short period. Therefore, pre-planning and having the ability to provide on-demand reinforcement, as required, is detrimental. For example, most paediatric trials would have a few enrolled participants, but what happens if three clinical trials simultaneously enrol fifteen to twenty participants each, not as initially planned for three to four participants? Is any pharmacy managed CT service prepared for such a change in intensity of work? The one I was managing was not! The service was unprepared to meet the demands of such a sudden and unanticipated increase in workload for two years per trial, followed by an additional two years for open-label extensions.

The healthcare ecosystem does not have mechanisms to react quickly enough to accommodate rapid or sudden workload increases. Additionally, CT service is a unique area requiring specialised knowledge, experience, and training. Thus, it is not as simple as moving general pharmacy staff from one area to help in another. GCP certification, CT-specific training, and signing on delegation logs for new or additional pharmacy staff is time-consuming. In practice, hurried staff training led to unsatisfactory performance and an unfavourable impact on the site's image.

Current staffing solutions of having a backup pharmacist on board appear sensible, but in practice, backup staff members lose perspective of trial work quickly if not involved regularly or frequently enough. Often, regardless of their limited confidence, knowledge, or experience, they deliver services under pressure and worry about the consequences later. Those are instances when IP error reporting, protocol deviations, regulatory non-compliance, or missing IPs are not dealt with immediately.

A more solid backup plan to meet service demands must be in place for the continuous provision of a high standard and sustainable paediatric pharmacy managed CT service. Staff reinforcement must be available and provided on short notice, as required. The potential for an increase in demands and capacity must be included in the strategic service planning.

TRACKING TOOLS

Excel spreadsheets or suitable software can be used. For accurate comparisons, use the same metrics for different tasks across all studies.

I used Excel and tracked the service's operational and financial performance. Both guide decision making, particularly when considering service expansion and growth in patient volume.

SERVICE OPERATIONAL PERFORMANCE TRACKING

What can we track? Why do we need to do so? What are the benefits?

The first measurement recordings took place when I started managing the service, as I had no data to shed light on its operational performance. What ignited my curiosity was some red flags: start and end dates on training and delegation logs revealed a frequent change of CT pharmacists; pharmacy folders appeared disorganised. At first glance, accountability logs showed incomplete entries; there were piles of unprocessed participant returns—all telltale signs of opportunities to improve the service.

So, establishing a baseline service status was essential. Without baseline data, it would have been unclear what improvements are required. I could not make informed decisions without a deeper understanding and richer insights. I almost always keep what is working well, as making ungrounded changes is not a successful strategy.

I started with asking questions to identify suitable metrics, which were used first for the measurement plan and then over time for tracking service performance:

- How many trials is the CT service managing in total?
- How many of them are investigator-driven?*
- How many are pharma sponsored?

- When did each CT commence?
- How many CTs do not have enrolled patients? Why?
- How many participants are enrolled per trial?
- How many visits per trial?
- How many items are dispensed per participant?
- How many months of IP supply per visit?
- Is trial enrolment open or closed?
- How many potential new participants may be enrolled?

Those are some questions that we can start with to identify metrics. They lead to other questions, allowing us to dig deeper. For example, the answers to future potential participant enrollment questions are better obtained directly from the PIs. They are happy to provide information about suitable prospective candidates. During my initial meetings with PIs and research team members, all those questions were asked, answered, and recorded. Within a few months, I had my database populated with more metrics than I originally had in mind. Individually and/or in combination, they have driven positive changes, improvements, and planning. *Paediatric pharmacy CT/research services cannot be managed effectively on good intentions only.*

*Note: institutional investigator-driven trials, by nature, are underfunded and often performed in kind, but their management is more time-consuming, especially if randomisation, IP accountability logs, blinding, sourcing of placebos, comparator treatments, and so on are required. While those research projects significantly contribute to children's pharmaceutical management, unfortunately, they may not lead to official market authorisation.

To determine which metrics to track, we need to keep getting back to the questions we are trying to answer and be clear about why and how we will use the answers to benefit the service.

Examples of further questions to help us with service planning include:

- At what stage is each trial?
- How many CTs are in the set up stage?
- When is each upcoming trial anticipated to start?
- What is each CT duration?
- How many CTs just started?
- How many are approaching the end?
- When is the enrolment closing? Has it already closed?
- How many new research projects are at the pre-feasibility visit stage?
- How many are in budget negotiation?
- Are the current resources adequate to support the requirements of the subsequent new trial?

The answers to the above questions and many others allow us to foresee better and plan additional participant visits and future services. Finding the correct answers is not difficult or time-consuming, as it may appear when it is done as part of our service management strategy. It is not about chasing information or questioning other team members relentlessly but about knowing what we do not know and ensuring we seek, capture, and record all relevant information.

Future service planning decisions are subject to answering questions that directly bear on our service, determining the metrics, and finally measuring and recording the data. An example is asking a CT technician to record the start and finish time of IP destruction of a certain number of kits, similarly, to sponsors requests during IP relabelling to record on a dedicated form the start and end time and the temperature throughout the task. Data gathered from comprehensive questions and metrics allow us to dig deeper into individual processes to identify and measure additional metrics for more informed decision making. Service operational performance tracking guided the decisions to support extra new trials while avoiding overcommitment. Participant safety and high quality data required for trial success cannot be disregarded, overlooked, or compromised.

SERVICE FINANCIAL TRACKING

Following a baseline assessment of the fees for pharmacy trial-related services and creating a financial tracking tool, the ongoing financial tracking shows the service operating income over time. The tracking tools should be suitable for individual service needs. For example, I used reminders for clinical trial agreements (CTAs) requiring amendments to jog my memory of when to approach sponsors. I used the date when the CTA was executed and the reasons for adjustments to guide the implementation time. Understandably, renegotiation of a recently executed agreement may not be possible without well-grounded reasons in the absence of protocol amendment, affecting pharmacy trial-related tasks. However, I have had a positive outcome with a renegotiation of a freshly negotiated/executed CTA by someone else. A sponsor's discretion and solid supporting data were the cornerstones for the positive outcome.

Some metric measurements used for tracking service operational performance can also determine service financial status and future economic projections or support funding of additional staffing.

Ultimately, all essential data initially collected for individual trials can be tracked at any point compared to previous ones for service financial performance assessment and for planning corrective steps to improve if required.

Including the names and contact details of PIs/SIs and CRCs in the tracking tool is helpful as a quick reference and to identify metrics for service improvements, which later can also be tracked. For example, the number of trials per CRC or PI can facilitate establishing appropriate communication frequency with individual teams while streamlining workflows.

ONGOING COLLECTION OF ROBUST DATA

'Everything that can be counted does not necessarily count; everything that counts cannot necessarily be counted'.

—ALBERT EINSTEIN

Ongoing collection of robust data for CT service improvements is in alignment with the legislative changes and incentives intended to encourage an ampler number and variety of paediatric CTs, as well as higher-quality research data. Any of the metrics I have listed below, and many more, can successfully be measured and used to drive desired changes:

- Number of dispensed items per month or another period
- Number of aseptic dispensing per month or another period
- Number of new trial protocols reviewed by CT pharmacist per month
- Ratio of PIs, CRCs, and monitors per one full-time equivalent CT pharmacist
- Number of successfully negotiated CTAs per month or another period
- Number of raised pharmacy invoices or service revenue per month or another period

- Number of site active research projects per quarter or another period
- Number of clinical visits, number of enrolled participants, and so on per period

My tracking of pre-selected metrics and occasionally reviewing and appropriately adjusting them, turned out to become a tried and proven sustainable practice.

Data-driven service operational performance changes had added benefits. Let us look at one example illustrating specific but targeted changes implemented to reduce the duration of pharmacy monitoring visits. Firstly, why was it essential for me? Because I was managing a busy CT service with little help of around two to two and a half hours per day. Time management was critical. Where and how I could gain time free of distractions and interactions became important questions. Most CRAs requested an average of two to three hours, which appeared like too much time is expended by monitoring visits. So, I decided to explore pharmacy monitoring visit duration as an operational indicator. The next logical step was to establish the average amount of time a monitor spends to verify the individual pharmacy source documents and IP reconciliation. I used the following metrics to guide the intended improvements:

1. Number of errors on logs
2. Number of shipments verified
3. Number of participant IP returns reconciled
4. Number and nature of clarifications

Let us focus on each one individually.

Metric number one, 'Number of errors on logs', is tightly related to the number of logs completed per clinical trial and the entries required.

What can be improved? How can it be done efficiently? I used post-dispensing reminders. Accurately completed logs guaranteed future time saving by not engaging in corrections. The next step to get me closer to my goal to reduce monitor visit duration was to merge participant visit IP prescriptions/orders with their accountability logs in individual plastic sleeves to shorten the verification process. It made a huge difference and resulted in an increased number of correct log entries and fewer omissions, which shortened the verification time.

Metric number two, 'Number of shipments verified'. A monitoring visit duration is dependent on the number of IP shipping documentation, their status, and the filing process. Verifying mixed shipping paperwork consumes monitors' and auditors' time as they have to match which papers belong to which shipment. Bundling each shipment's paperwork together and filling them by date of receipt significantly reduced verification time.

Metric number three, 'Number of participant IP returns reconciled'. Counting and verifying the accurateness of IPs returned by participants is another time-consuming task independent of the monitor's experience. Each participant's returns correctly counted and entered in logs were placed in a separate plastic bag, which streamlined the process. As a result, the monitors performed quicker IP reconciliation, and I had fewer disruptions for clarification. The outcome—all monitoring visits were notably shortened, and I freed myself time for other service improvements.

Lastly, I want to comment on the benefits of service and processes tracking. What are the justifications of engagement? Does tracking contribute towards *Evolving the Dinosaur*?

Having immediate access to service performance and financial data is fundamental for further service improvements. To name a few:

- Allows assessing pharmacy CT service capacity to support forthcoming, new trials without compromising a patient's safety, quality services, and data integrity.
- Allows proactive, preventive, and corrective measures to be taken promptly, including improved legislative and protocol compliance.
- Financial tracking helps future financial service projections. They are rarely precise due to many variables, but they are a valuable guide.

CT pharmacist tasks and overall responsibility may differ between hospitals based on the research service set up. However, they balance multiple responsibilities simultaneously with the exponential increase in workloads due to the growing demand for their services.

Data-driven changes, measuring and tracking, provides a real-time check on change progress and adjustments, fast-tracking the pharmacy CT services to greater strategic management, efficiencies, and improved operations, all contributing towards *Evolving the Dinosaur*.

The Future

'If you cannot do great things, do small things in a great way'.

—NAPOLEON HILL

Now that we are nearing the end, I want to thank you for making it through the book.

All effort has been made to bridge the understanding gap of CT pharmacists' pain points to their root causes. However, those specific challenges have not been previously explored, addressed or attempted to be solved, as stakeholders involved in paediatric trials cannot solve problems, they are not aware of or know how others are impacted.

Clinical trial implementation cannot be fully understood if all team member contributions are not considered together as a whole. A successful execution does not belong to one specific individual or group—PI, clinical research coordinator, pharmacist, CRA, CRO, sponsor, or EC/IRB—but to everyone involved and relies on their expertise, input, and collaboration. Paediatric drug development challenges cannot be managed if the individual stakeholders' function in silos because we cannot be experts in everything.

Teamwork and inter-professional collaboration are the foundation for consistently refining participant-centred care and services to attain high quality clinical trial data. They are also the basis for evaluation and continual improvements of the way we do things.

CT pharmacists may have innovative ideas or an intrapreneurial mindset, medication safety strategies, or quality improvement and change management initiatives; however, acting on them depends not only on their ability but on other stakeholders' understanding, commitment, and support. The nature of their work and the way it is organised does not usually support engagements with clinical research teams or external stakeholders away from the pharmacy. They do not usually have flexibility built into their day-to-day work schedules to do so. It is anticipated that they engage to various degrees but without formal expectations. Without dedicated time and institutional support, CT/research pharmacists cannot turn their innovative ideas into action. All of this limits their beneficial impact. Additionally, it limits their ability to ascertain their authentic contributions and focus on the bigger picture rather than on the daily trial related tasks only.

In this book, I did not attempt to address or solve all issues encountered during trial implementation but to highlight some of their root causes I believe persist needlessly.

Care and effort have been made to explore the consequences of various tenacious issues and the benefits if resolved. My long years of experience in paediatric clinical trials, medication safety, and the front line of clinical practice have served in working out practical solutions, as presented throughout the book.

Learning from the past, from others—from their successes and failures—is critical for future success. Even with its complexities, challenges, and mountains of obstacles, paediatric clinical research's path forward involves better understanding and consideration of all team members' and stakeholders' contributions, collaboration, commitment, and working in synergy. Commitment comes about when those impacted start genuinely working in a new way, whether through new processes, new systems, or new behaviours.

Peter Drucker, a US management consultant, once said, 'The best way to predict the future is to create it'.

I dedicate the conclusion to the future *Evolving the Dinosaur*. The next crucial move in the paediatric research evolution is up to sponsors, CROs, PIs, paediatric researchers, pharmacists, patient advocacy groups, and ethical committees to create a more supportive and welcoming environment, with the inclusion of diverse expertise during the various drug development stages.

The answers to the following questions are explored in these last pages in no specific order of importance: What does the future of paediatric clinical trial pharmacists look like? What expanded practice roles might they have? Why should sponsors/CROs work closely with the pharmaceutical experts?

EXPERIENTIAL BEST PRACTICE FOR SITE INITIATION VISITS (SIVS)

I leveraged SIVs to accomplish two critical tasks—to meet the trial team members, CRAs, and other external attendees and to assess their commitment to future collaboration. Secondly, to address the issues, if any, surrounding the pharmaceutical portion of the trial. The protocol presentations usually generate insightful discussions and clarifications of expressed concerns—all of which are remarkably useful to pharmacists. SIVs is the place and the time for pharmacy-specific issues, concerns, safety risks, and investigational product logistics to be raised for discussion or clarification. Essentially, all internal and external participants should use the SIV to become better acquainted and pave the way for team success, as the site will succeed or fail as a team. The most satisfying experiences have been when all involved in the trial have been aligned and teamed up towards the common goal: a successful administration. In healthcare, collaboration and *coordination,* or working towards the same goal, and *cooperation,* or contributing to the team—coincide. Also, the decision making is shared, based on communication, negotiation, and respectful power balance. The relationships between principal investigators, pharmacists, and research coordinators in a hospital setting are cultivated over time, and all members work equitably together.

I invite sponsors, CROs and other drug development stakeholders to embrace site teams' diversity of knowledge, skills, and experience in paediatrics and align goals, resources, and commitment towards more effective multistakeholder collaboration to make future paediatric research more efficient, leading to the labelling of more new treatments.

The COVID-19 pandemic added new challenges to the already burdened paediatric research community. Shifting to virtual clinical trials requires a more integrated approach than ever across all stakeholders. A comprehensive evaluation of risks versus benefits; participant convenience versus their needs and safety; and what's best for participants versus best for trial data for regulatory approval requires sponsors, CROs, and sites to further diversify and balance expertise exchange to deliver quality implementation and results while concurrently managing risks.

COUNSELLING TO CLINICAL TRIAL PARTICIPANTS AND MONITORING IP COMPLIANCE

Pharmacists have a substantial positive impact on patient care and therapeutic outcomes through effective counselling. They also provide information to other healthcare professionals on the safe, effective, and efficient use of medicines. This professional skill is underutilised in the clinical trials' area. It continues to be a delegated task by PIs and not standardised, instead of being a routine practice.

With luck, future changes will lead to official allocation to the pharmacists. Research reveals a compliance rate of 98 per cent for participants who received IP counselling from pharmacists compared to 76 per cent for those who did not. Also, participant compliance rates declined with an increase in dosing frequency, and the decrease was more significant (from 81 per cent to 67 per cent) when a CT pharmacist had not counselled participants.[24]

However, for now, CT pharmacists must keep up their high level of knowledge and credibility in providing effective and comprehensive trial and investigational product information to participants and their caregivers, medical and nursing staff, and researchers, according to the target audience and in conjunction with the PIs.

CLINICAL TRIAL DESIGN, METHODOLOGY, AND PROTOCOL REVIEW

CT pharmacists' early input into the pharmaceutical part of new paediatric clinical trials is essential. For example, unnecessarily complicated protocols, data collection tools, training materials, or information resources can create confusion and delay due to the lack of a direct CT pharmacist-sponsor/CRO feedback loop or not having an immediate remedial action plan in place. Therefore, adopting new direct communication and collaboration approaches is much anticipated.

Experienced paediatric pharmacists can have valuable input reviewing new protocols and making recommendations for modifications, as required. Prompt resolution of IP-related issues can prevent poorly designed trials to start in the first place. Amendments of approved protocols are time-consuming and drive costs up, compared to identifying and rectifying issues early and paving the way for a trouble-free research project approval and execution.

Paediatric CT pharmacists' expertise can be outsourced through external pharmacist consultants/advisors to provide expert or second opinion on the pharmaceutical aspects of new paediatric trials by assessing the design and methodology, the choice of comparator drugs, blinding, formulations, and likely administration issues, as well as handling safety risks.

Information on IPs interactions with milk and food (typical for infants' and children's diets) needs to become a standard practice and be included in all new CT protocols and pharmacy manuals.

ADVERSE DRUG REACTION REPORTING

Safety reporting is the PI's responsibility. However, CT pharmacists ensure participants' safety is not overlooked or mismanaged by other less experienced research team members.

For example, when appropriate, they can request that the first dose of a new IP is administered at the hospital, in an appropriate, safe area, and the participant is monitored to avoid complications with an immediate adverse reaction post the first dose.

Adverse drug reactions in paediatric patients require greater vigilance because they are more susceptible. Future, more active and standardised involvement of research pharmacists in monitoring and reporting adverse reactions would enhance participants safety.

Awareness of the weight of pharmacovigilance in children, ADR detection and reporting, in addition to establishing *plans for long-term safety monitoring*, should be extended to the site's team members and other external stakeholders.

THERAPEUTIC DRUG MONITORING (TDM)

TDM for investigational products is performed if required by the trial protocol, but CT pharmacist's do not routinely see participants, and the extent of their clinical input to review or follow-up on test results is not established. That is another role that CT pharmacists should perform in their professional capacity in the future.

ADVISING ON CLINICAL TRIAL REGULATORY ASPECTS

Unfortunately, universally not many CT pharmacists are experienced in local or global clinical trial regulatory affairs. It is a specialised role rather than a standardised routine research pharmacist's practice. From experience, very few sponsors would consult the CT pharmacy about regulatory issues, as it is the domain of the hospital's research governance offices and ECs/IRBs. While there are inter-institutional and international variances in practice, CT pharmacists should play a more active role in reviewing investigational product materials, labelling, batch records, specification sheets, and test methods for compliance with applicable regulations and policies. In addition, it would be beneficial for them to better understand the aspects of product development, manufacturing practices, regulations, and approval processes.

EXTERNAL PAEDIATRIC PHARMACISTS: CONSULTANTS/ ADVISORS

Research pharmacists play an irreplaceable role throughout clinical trial implementation, and their multidimensional input is distinct. Managing a paediatric pharmacy CT service means new challenges are expected every day and a sense of achievement when everything is resolved successfully. Historically, many hospital pharmacies have started managing clinical trials as an 'add on' to their various clinical and non-clinical tasks.

The growing demand for paediatric pharmacy trial-related services by pharma companies and institutional researchers continuously necessitated *extra pharmacists working hours* to be redirected towards the area, or even a *dedicated team of CT pharmacists and technicians* to work in this rapidly expanding area of pharmacy specialty.

The increasing numbers and complexity of paediatric CTs, coupled with the requirements for high standard research, further increase the demand for well-trained paediatric research personnel. The imbalance between the increased demand and a limited supply of trained paediatric staff further complicates and worsens the situation.

Ideally, a comprehensive assessment of a new trial's requirements against the pharmacy's physical and human resources capacity is performed before endorsing support. However, the reality is that pharmacists would rather be supportive than perceived as unaccommodating despite a staffing deficit; thus, they may take on board much more than they can safely manage. Also, knowing the importance of clinical research and appreciating the growing need for safe and evidence-based therapies for infants and children makes it harder to turn down new trials. As it happens, pharmacy CT services easily overcommit to support too many projects, without having the actual resources, resulting in overburdened, anxious, and fatigued pharmacists due to excessive workload and pressure. Unfortunately, those are the times when practice standards and medication safety can be inadvertently compromised.

The pharmacy clinical trial area is not very attractive for young pharmacists, attributable to limited career progression. In my humble opinion, this area of the pharmacy profession would benefit from *uplift* to become more appealing to newly graduated pharmacists while retaining experienced ones.

Time constraints, lack of flexibility, and limited support are the main reasons CT pharmacists do not turn their innovative ideas into action or do not participate in the new trial approval decision-making process, to name a few. Would a young and inexperienced pharmacist be up for such insurmountable challenges? Can a new practitioner who may lack professional and social intelligence maneuver internal roadblocks and various superiors to succeed? Maybe in the future, we will see intrapreneurship-structured teaching included in the pharmacy curriculum and postgraduate residencies or offered as continuing education or through internally/externally funded coaching. It could turn out to be a well-justified return on investment.

I attempted to provide readers with a detailed overview of the paediatric CT/research pharmacist contributions and challenges and how they can turn them into opportunities for improvements. I envision future pharmacy practitioners broadening their involvement since their specialised training and unique expertise are underutilised in paediatric research.

Additionally, CT/research pharmacists should assume total educational responsibilities over the trial pharmaceuticals to break off some misguided training practices driven by tradition as an excuse.

A recent editorial titled 'Hero Clinical Pharmacists and the COVID-19 Pandemic: Overworked and Overlooked' re-established that hospitals, academic health centres, and healthcare providers acknowledge pharmacists as valued team members, stating, 'This knowledge has not always been translated to the public, the news media, and politicians'.[25] I am in total agreement that in the paediatric clinical research ecosystem, this knowledge is not yet translated to sponsors, CROs, and other external stakeholders.

Externally commissioned paediatric research pharmacists as consultants/advisors/coaches can be very resourceful during

SIVs and trial implementation to guide, coach, and motivate underperforming sites due to their know-how to combine their insider perspectives with the sites' perspectives for reaching the best-personalised solutions.

Usually, paediatric hospital pharmacy departments integrate their best practice with established governance and medication handling, according to local legislative acts, health policies, directives, standards, and guidelines relevant to medication handling.

Applying the best paediatric clinical practices in clinical trials management is in line with participant safety, considering protocol's complexity, dosing regimens, and lack of complete information on IPs' adverse event profiles. In addition, future standardising of the best clinical trial practices across clinical trials and clinical sites can offer an additional layer of participant safeguarding.

WHAT CAN WE LEARN FROM THE PAPER-BASED PAEDIATRIC CLINICAL TRIALS?

COVID-19 has brought to light that paper-based clinical trials cannot support the future.

Sponsors and CROs dived enthusiastically into implementing digital platforms/software and various virtual solutions initially designed to suit their own needs and then forced them on sites, regardless of their functionality and practicality. However, are those virtual solutions a quantum leap or a digital transformation of former practices? What has changed if new technologies make conducting trials easier but shift work and responsibility between stakeholders?

Paediatric research challenges continue to be managed in silos. For example, the people who write protocols and create pharmacy manuals and data collection tools do not meet trial participants, clinical trial pharmacists, or research teams. Meanwhile, site teams, who look after participants, do not write protocols or pharmacy manuals, or meet the people who do.

The way forward? Why not use the lessons learned from paper based CTs to gather the proper requirements to design the right tools for the right people in the context of individual circumstances, needs, contributions, and feedback?

This book is a snapshot of how a paediatric pharmacy CT service implemented its change, measure, and track system to gather requirements. In addition, it outlined how sponsors and CROs can collaborate and partner with pharmacy CT services to integrate this know-how into future virtual multifunctional research portal features.

These use cases can be utilised to create integrated solutions that weigh in on:

1. Comprehensive evaluation of risks versus benefits
2. Participant convenience versus their needs and safety
3. What is best for patients versus what is best for the trial data for regulatory approval while maintaining high-quality patient-centred services, compliance, and risk management.

The COVID-19 pandemic created new additional challenges to those discussed at the beginning of the book. Sponsors, CROs, and sites need to deliver virtual high quality care and services, while managing risks in the context of individual participant/family circumstances. The pandemic also created new possibilities, but one solution does not fit all, especially for global clinical trials, as the COVID-19 impact and response have varied from country to country.

Currently, the focus is on virtual medicine/telemedicine, which sounds exciting for most of us who are comfortable with technology and open to engaging virtually, but there are stacks of unanswered questions and issues yet to be contemplated. For example, do the solutions we design meet the needs of the highly variable paediatric patient base? Practical solutions will need to consider whether we can measure, report, and track the impact of virtual interventions on the widely variable demographics of trial participants, technology comfort, family lifestyle, and logistics while maintaining the provision of quality patient-centred care, compliance, and managing the risks.

Sponsors, more than ever, would require diverse expertise and partnerships with other stakeholders for a successful shift to virtual healthcare.

FINAL THOUGHTS

The intention of sharing my success with *Evolving the Dinosaur* and the lessons learned is to help others get ahead faster by applying them to individual needs. Also, to equip others with the tools and confidence for rapid and sustainable growth. Adopting a stance for change and an intrapreneurial mindset was just as necessary during the journey.

I have put much work into researching the fundamental metrics for swift but safe change management. I conclude that the central key performance indicators (KPIs) fall into operations, research teams, financials, and service growth. We cannot improve if we do not measure; if we do not track, we cannot assess our progress or lack of it.

Evolving the Dinosaur offers various clinical research stakeholders an opportunity to get familiar with pharmacy CT service and pharmacist practices, inputs, challenges, and opportunities for improvement.

Sponsors and CROs can use the book as an appeal for stronger collaboration towards finding the best mitigation strategies to minimise IP safety risks and improve pharmacy manuals, information resources, and data collection tools.

It is expected that more medication safety initiatives are incorporated in paediatric protocols, interactive response technologies, and better alignment of IP names, packaging, and labelling with medication safety principles.

Understandably, drug development stakeholders are predominantly focused on IP safety profiles and clinical efficacy. Professionally, pharmacists are best versed with medication safety principles; thus, naturally, they have taken over IP safety management and error mitigation at the site level throughout clinical trial execution. However, future shared understanding of the problems and better alignment around goals, commitment, and collaboration is the way forward. For example, the limited regulatory guidance on IP names, labelling, and packaging to promote safety can be compensated by outsourcing and engaging external paediatric consultants/advisor pharmacists to guide the way pragmatically.

Medication safety has been heavily incorporated into my daily work over the last twenty years. I used its principles successfully in my clinical trial practice as well. However, future improvements in this area require multistakeholder collaboration and standardised strategic planning to identify specific risks and formulate feasible solutions.

Paediatric clinical research stakeholders got more familiar with why early and direct involvement of site CT pharmacists is crucial. The detailed insights of their unique positioning, medication safety management, and pain point causes are genuine attempts to inspire future improvements.

Institutional, pharmacy, and research leaders/managers have been made aware of employees with an intrapreneurial mindset who require incentives, encouragement, and support. Meanwhile, intrapreneurs will continue to enhance the delivery of health care services and improve the quality of patient care. However, hospitals and health institutions cannot rely on a few lonely intrapreneurs to change the system.

I wish *Evolving of the Dinosaur* gets across to as many paediatric clinical research stakeholders as possible. For example, external stakeholders may not be aware or considered that frequently trial participants are hospital and pharmacy patients; the pharmacists know those patients from previous hospital admissions or regularly dispense their usual medications and already have established trust. For the same reason, pharmacists are routinely the first point of inquiry about investigational products or clinical trials; thus, better information resources are directly related to enhanced participants' trial journeys.

While sponsors, CROs, and sites throughout COVID-19 are adopting multifunctional research portals and adjusting towards remote operations by enabling virtual investigator meetings, site initiation visits, remote document management, e-learning, and so on, the CT pharmacists may have been left out again due to the gap of awareness of their input beyond IP management and dispensing. In addition, a lack of a direct feedback loop of what the CT pharmacist needs are and how they can be met can lead to lost initiatives when clinical site pharmacists are provided with unsuitable online self-services, or they do not have the time to use them.

Thank you again for choosing *Evolving the Dinosaur*! Every effort was made to ensure it is full of as much insightful information as possible.

If you found this book valuable somehow, please consider recommending it to anyone else who may benefit from it, too.

'If you want something new, you have to stop doing something old'.

—PETER DRUCKER

Further Reading

ASHP Guidelines for the Management of Investigational Drug Products. Published by the American Society of Health-System Pharmacists November 8, 2017. https://www.ashp.org/-/media/assets/policy-guidelines/docs/guidelines/management-investigational-drug-products.ashx.

HOPA Investigational Drug Service Best Practice Standards by Sapna R. Amin, Joyce E. Lee, et al. Published by the Hematology/Oncology Pharmacists Association in 2014. https://www.hoparx.org/images/hopa/resource-library/professional-tools/HOPA16_IDS_Guidelines.pdf.

How to Identify and Manage 'Problem' Excipients in Medicines for Children by Sara Arthur and Anna Burgess. Published by *The Pharmaceutical Journal* in July 2017. https://pharmaceutical-journal.com/article/ld/how-to-identify-and-manage-problem-excipients-in-medicines-for-children.

Recommendations for Terminology, Abbreviations and Symbols Used in Medicines Documentation by the Australian Commission on Safety and Quality in Health Care. December 2016. https://www.safetyandquality.gov.au/sites/default/files/migrated/Recommendations-for-terminology-abbreviations-and-symbols-used-in-medicines-December-2016.pdf.

Paediatric Pharmacokinetics: Key Considerations by Hannah Katherine Batchelor and John Francis Marriott. Published by the *British Journal of Clinical Pharmacology* in October 2013. Accessed June 23, 2020. DOI: 10.1111/bcp.12267.

Medication Safety in Clinical Trials: Role of the Pharmacist in Optimizing Practice, Collaboration, and Education to Reduce Errors by Jamie N. Brown, Sara R. Britnell, Andrew P. Stivers, and Jennifer L. Cruz. Published by *The Yale Journal of Biology and Medicine* in 2017. PMID: 28356900.

Enhancing the Pediatric Drug Development Framework to Deliver Better Pediatric Therapies Tomorrow by Christina Bucci-Rechtweg. Published by *Clinical Therapeutics* in 2017. DOI: 10.1016/j.clinthera.2017.07.043.

Challenges in Paediatric Clinical Trials: How to Make It Feasible by G. Chiaruttini, M. Felisi and D. Bonifazi. Published by Intech in June 2018. Accessed January 14, 2020. https://www.intechopen.com/books/the-management-of-clinical-trials/challenges-in-paediatric-clinical-trials-how-to-make-it-feasible.

Safety Risks with Investigational Drugs: Pharmacy Practices and Perceptions in the Veterans' Affairs Health System by Jennifer L. Cruz and Jamie N. Brown. Published by *Therapeutic Advances in Drug Safety* in 2015. DOI: 10.1177/2042098615584924.

Neonates Exposed to Excipients: Concern about Safety by Laura Cuzzolin. Published by *Journal of Pediatric and Neonatal Individualized Medicine* in 2018. DOI: 10.7363/070112.

Department of Veterans Affairs: Investigational Drugs and Supplies. VHA Handbook 1108.04. http://www.va.gov/vhapublications/ViewPublication.asp?pub_ID=2497.

SIMulation of Medication Error Induced by Clinical Trial drug Labeling: The SIMME-CT Study by Cecile Dollinger, Vérane Schwiertz, Laura Sarfati, Chloé Gourc-Berthod, Marie-Gabrielle Guédat, Céline Alloux, et al. Published by *International Journal for Quality in Health Care* in 2016. DOI: 10.1093/intqhc/mzw025.

10-Year Report to the European Commission by the European Medicines Agency and its Paediatric Committee. Published October 2016. EMA/231225/2015.

Guideline on Pharmaceutical Development of Medicines for Paediatric Use. Published by European Medicines Agency in 2013. http://www.ema.europa.eu/docs/en_GB/document_library/Scientific_guideline/2013/07/WC500147002.pdf.

Product Codes and Product Code Builder. Published by the Food and Drug Administration, last updated May 2018. https://www.fda.gov/industry/import-program-resources/product-codes-and-product-code-builder.

Food and Drug Administration: Investigational New Drug Application. Code of Federal Regulations, Title 21, Chapter 312. https://www.accessdata.fda.gov/scripts/cdrh/cfdocs/cfCFR/CFRSearch.cfm?CFRPart=312.

Food and Drug Administration: Pediatrics. Accessed August 25, 2019. https://www.fda.gov/science-research/science-and-research-special-topics/pediatrics.

Report: Survey of Current Guidance for Child Health Clinical Trials by F. N. J. Frakking, J. H. van der Lee, T. P. Klassen, M. Offinga. Compiled for the StaR-Child Health Group of the World Health Organization. Accessed August 2019. https://www.who.int/childmedicines/publications/GUIDANCECHILDHEALTH.pdf.

Development of sensory information processing—the ontogenesis of opioid binding sites in nociceptive afferents and their significance in the clinical setting by E. Freye. Published by *Acta Anaesthesiologica Scandinavica* (Suppl.) in 1996.

Reducing the potential for mistakes with investigational drugs by Matthew Grissinger. Published by *P&T* in 2011. PMID: 21572761.

The Role of Clinical Trials Pharmacist in Study Medication Adherence by Eugenia Hong. Paper given at 7th Pharmacovigilance & Pharmaceutical Industry conference in 2016. DOI: 10.4172/2329-6887.C1.019.

Preventing Medication Errors by Institute of Medicine. Edited by Linda R. Cronenwett, J. Lyle Bootman, Julie Wolcott, and Philip Aspden. Published by National Academies Press in 2007.

Guidelines for Safe Electronic Communication of Medication Information by the Institute for Safe Medication Practices (IMSP). Published January 16, 2019. https://www.ismp.org/resources/guidelines-safe-electronic-communication-medication-information.

Guidelines for Standard Order Sets by the Institute for Safe Medication Practices. Published January 12, 2010. https://www.ismp.org/guidelines/standard-order-sets.

Investigational Drugs: Product-Related Issues Pose Significant Challenges (Part I) by the Institute for Safe Medication Practices. Published April 19, 2018. https://www.ismp.org/resources/investigational-drugs-product-related-issues-pose-significant-challenges-part-i.

Investigational Drugs: Strategies for Sponsors, FDA, and Clinical Sites to Prevent Product-Related Errors (Part II) by the Institute for Safe Medication Practices. Published May 3, 2018. https://www.ismp.org/resources/investigational-drugs-strategies-sponsors-fda-and-clinical-sites-prevent-product-related.

List of Error-Prone Abbreviations by the Institute for Safe Medication Practices. Published Februrary 5, 2021. https://www.ismp.org/recommendations/error-prone-abbreviations-list.

Product-Related Issues Make Error Potential Enormous with Investigational Drugs by the Institute for Safe Medication Practices. Published November 2007. https://www.ismp.org/resources/product-related-issues-make-error-potential-enormous-investigational-drugs.

Side Tracks on the Safety Express. Interruptions Lead to Errors and Unfinished… Wait, What Was I Doing? by the Institute for Safe Medication Practices. Published November 19, 2012. https://www.ismp.org/resources/side-tracks-safety-express-interruptions-lead-errors-and-unfinished-wait-what-was-i-doing.

Participation of a Coordinating Center Pharmacy in a Multicenter International Study by Jihyun Esther Jeon, Janet Mighty, Karen Lane, Nichol McBee, Ryan Majkowski, Steven Mayo, and Daniel Hanley. Published by *American Journal of Health-System Pharmacy* in 2016. DOI: 10.2146/ajhp150849.

ASHP Guidelines for the Management of Investigational Drug Products by Stephen C. Kay, Darlette G. Luke, and Helen R. Tamer. Published by *American Journal of Health-System Pharmacy* in 2018. DOI: 10.2147/ajhp170812.

Developmental Pharmacokinetics in Pediatric Populations by Hong Lu and Sara Rosenbaum. Published by *The Journal of Pediatric Pharmacology and Therapeutics* in October 2014. Accessed June 23, 2020. DOI: 10.5863/1551-6776-19.4.262.

Clinical Drug Trials by Amy Mason. Published by *Pediatrics in Review* in March 2018. DOI: 10.1542/pir.2016-0230.

Pediatrics by Milap C. Nahata and Carol Taketomo. Chapter 6 of *Pharmacotherapy: A Pathophysiologic Approach, 10th edition*, edited by Joseph T. DiPiro, Robert L. Talbert, Gary C. Yee, Gary R. Matzke, Barbara G. Wells, and L. Michael Posey. Published by McGraw-Hill in 2017. https://accesspharmacy.mhmedical.com/content.aspx?bookid=1861&sectionid=146077859.

Kinetics and Dynamics of Postoperative Intravenous Morphine in Children by Klaus T. Olkkola, Eeva-Liisa Maunuksela, Reijo Korpela and Per H. Rosenberg. Published by Clinical Pharmacology and Therapeutics in 1988. DOI: 10.1038/cipt.1988/127.

Clinical research: ASHP Guidelines and Future Directions for Pharmacists by Marjorie Shaw Phillips. Published by *American Journal of Health-System Pharmacy* in February 1999. DOI: 10.1093/ajhp/56.4.344.

Dispensing Investigational Drugs: Regulatory Issues and the Role of the Investigational Drug Service by Nadine Shehab and Helen Tamer. Published by *American Journal of Health-System Pharmacy* in 2004. DOI: 10.1093/ajhp/61.18.1882.

Pharmacist-Prepared Dispensing Guidelines for Drugs Used in Clinical Research by Rivka Siden, Helen R. Tamer, Amy J. Skyles, Susan Weadock, and Kimberly Redic. Published by *American Journal of Health-System Pharmacy* in 2012. DOI: 10.2146/ajhp110082.

Pediatric Product Development in the U.S. by Jean Temeck. Published by the *Food and Drug Administration, Office of Pediatric Therapeutics* in November 2010. Accessed June 23, 2020. https://www.fda.gov/media/81290/download.

Developmental Changes in Pharmacokinetics and Pharmacodynamics by John van den Anker, Michael D. Reed, Karel Allegaert, and Gregory L. Kearns. Published by *The Journal of Clinical Pharmacology* in 2018. Accessed August 27, 2019. DOI: 10.1002/jcph.1284.

World Health Organisation: Promoting Safety of Medicines for Children. Accessed June 23, 2020. https://www.who.int/medicines/publications/essentialmedicines/Promotion_safe_med_childrens.pdf.

Liquid Medication Dosing Errors in Children: Role of Provider Counseling Strategies by H. Shonna Yin, Benard P. Dreye, Hannah A. Moreira, Linda van Schaick, Luis Rodriguez et al. Published by *Academic Pediatrics* in 2014. DOI: 10.1016/j.acap.2014.01.003.

National Survey of Pharmacy-Coordinated Investigational Drug Services by L. M. Young, C. M. Haakenson, J. H. Weber, and T. J. Tosch. Published by *American Journal of Hospital Pharmacy* in 1984. PMID: 6496514.

Kinetics and dynamics of postoperative intravenous morphine in children by K.T. Olkkola, E.L. Maunuksela, R. Korpela, and P.H. Rosenberg. Published in *Clinical Pharmacology and Therapeutics* 44 (1988): 128-136.

Consequences of Individual's Fit at Work: A Meta-Analysis of Person–Job, Person–Organization, Person–Group, and Person–Supervisor Fit by A. L. Kristof-Brown, R. D. Zimmerman, and E. C. Johnson. Published by *Personnel Psychology*, 58 (2005): 281–342.

Appendix

INSTRUCTIONS FOR DISPERSING IP (DISPERSIBLE TABLET) IN AN ORAL SYRINGE

CT Participant Name: ______________________ **MRN:** _________

CT Name/No.: ____

Date: ____

Current Dose: ______ times per day

For the preparation of **each dose**, you will need:

- IP name______________ strength______________ disp. tab
- No of tabs ___________ = (___________ mg/microgram)
- 1 × size syringe, e.g., 5 mL or 10 mL
- 1 × syringe cap
- Water

INSTRUCTIONS

1. Pull plunger out of the syringe.
2. Place dispersible tablet(s) into the syringe barrel.
3. Replace plunger.
4. Draw up ___ mL of water into the syringe with the dispersible tablet(s) plus 1–2 mL of air, without pulling out the plunger.
5. Put syringe cap on syringe tip.
6. Shake the syringe gently for X seconds/minutes to allow the tablet to disperse.
7. Give the contents of the entire syringe directly into your child's mouth within X minutes/hours of dose preparation. Note: may/may not be given via nasogastric tube.
8. Draw up a further ___ mL of water into the syringe and gently shake the syringe to disperse or wash out any IP residue left in the syringe.
9. Give the contents of the entire syringe directly into your child's mouth.

The IP dose should be followed by a drink of at least ___ mL of water to wash down any medication residue in the mouth.

NEW CLINICAL TRIAL QUESTIONNAIRE

- Multicentre/single centre?
- Open label/single or double-blinded?
- Phase?
- International?
- Name of sponsor
- Name of CRO
- CRA contact name, email, and phone number (if known)
- Expected frequency of face to face monitoring visits

- Anticipated remote/off site monitoring frequency (via phone or other medium)
- Dispensing schedule e.g., D1, D15, W4, W8, W16... (D = day, W = week)
- Number of IP dispensing visits per patient
- Expected length of trial
- Expected first patient's first visit date (FPFV)
- Expected first patient's first last visit date (FPLV)
- Expected last patient's first visit date (LPFV)
- Expected last patient's last visit date (LPLV)
- Target number of patients to be enrolled at site
- Is IRT required for both receiving IP and participant returns? (Yes/No)
- Are there any randomisation requirements?
- What are the CT pharmacy blinding requirements, if any?
- Packaging and shipments (how IPs would be packaged: e.g., single bottles, kits)
- What is the size of a single container? (for storage assessment)
- How many bottles/kits/etc. will be in the first shipment?
- Are subsequent IP shipments auto-generated post each participant's dispensing?
- Is ongoing supply of ancillary items automatic or manual (reordering by CT pharmacist)?
- Special requirements and other comments:
- **Note!** This is not a comprehensive list of questions.

Once all information is gathered and assessed, the individual fees are calculated, and the prepared budget is submitted to the sponsor or delegate for review, approval, and signature.

CUSTOMISABLE CLINICAL TRIAL SUMMARY TEMPLATE

CUSTOMISABLE **CT SUMMARY** TEMPLATE

Hospital/Health Service Name:

CT Service/Pharmacy Department

Pediatric CT Summary

VERSION	DATE

Clinical Trial Name: ______________________________

Clinical Trial Protocol Number/Short Name: ______________________

Version: ______________ Date: ______________

Pharmacy Manual: ______________________________

Version: ______________ Date: ______________

Ethics/IRB Approval Number: __________________________

Principal Investigator (PI) Name: ________________________

Clinical Research Coordinator (CRC) Name: ____________________

Funding/Sponsors Name: ____________________________

Site Contact Team Members Contact Details:

CT Team Members	Email	Phone/Mobile	Pager/ Ext No.
PI			
Sub Investigator			
CRC			

CT overview: Provide a brief description.

Investigational product (IP): Provide dosing and administration information, dispensing per visit, number of visits, dosing, dispensing errors reporting, and IP complaints reporting.

IP storage: Explain conditions, temperature monitoring, and site pharmacy location, if required.

Ongoing ordering: If manual, provide supplier's name/email/ phone number +/– other required information.

IP receipt: Explain what actions must be taken and what accountability logs need to be completed.

Ancillary items: Explain what and when is provided to study participants and ongoing supply.

CT design: Provide a brief description.

CT prescription (Rx)/order: Explain when it is completed and how it is delivered to a CT pharmacy.

Dispensing: Describe applicable site-specific dispensing process and pharmacy dispensing software.

IP labelling: Administration instructions must be consistent with protocol, original IP containers, and the trial prescription order.

Caution statement: The label must state that the IP is for clinical research purposes only or similar. For the USA: 'Caution: New Drug—Limited by federal law to investigational use'. Also, include a reminder to return all unused, partially used, and empty containers to pharmacy.

Auxiliary labels: If required (e.g., teratogenic IP + handling precautions).

Sample dispensing label: Affix it in provided space below.

Short CT Name
IP name, strength, dose form, and quantity supplied
Directions for use, frequency, and dose
Participant's name and their study number
Date of dispensing and CT pharmacist initials
IP batch/lot number and container/kit number
Pharmacy name, address, and telephone number
Prescriber's (PI/SI) name
Storage directions
'Keep out of reach of children'

Dispensing labels must comply with local legislation and regulations, with institutional policies and procedures, as well as with the protocol requirements. The institution's contact information and PI's name are also required.

Special instructions or auxiliary labels must be provided, too. For example, food intake recommendations, storage conditions, and expiry date, if shelf life is different post opening—discard X days post opening (date opened __/__/__).

IP Accountability Logs (IPALs): Specify how many IPALs need to be completed—master IP accountability log and individual or participant IP accountability log or a single log. Describe how it is to be completed, manually, electronically, or both.

Storage of dispensed IPs: Describe IP storage and location of dispensed products before collection from CT pharmacy.

Collection of dispensed IPs: Describe who is authorised to collect dispensed IPs and any other necessary steps, for example, if collector needs to sign the prescription to acknowledge receipt of the clinical trial items.

Counselling on IP administration: Specify who counsels the participants and provide a brief description and the important points.

Direct to patient IP shipping: Describe the process.

IP returns by trial participants: Describe the process of manipulating returns, safety precautions and whether counting, weighing, or measuring volume of liquid products is required; what forms/logs need to be completed. Define if electronic recording is required and when it is performed: before or after being reconciled by the CRA and place of storage. For example, no IP returns by participants for this study: participant's compliance measured by assessment of patients' clinical response and study diaries. Not performed by CT pharmacists.

Best practice is to prepare a clinical trial customised summary that balances rigor and practicality and promotes effectiveness and participant safety.

CUSTOMISABLE CLINICAL TRIAL PRESCRIPTION TEMPLATE

CT PRESCRIPTION TEMPLATE

EXAMPLE Rx FOR INJECTABLE IP VIALS

ALLERGY

CT Prescription

For Hospital Use Only

CT name: ____

____

CT short name: ____

Ethics/IRB Approval No.: ____________

Principal investigator: Dr./Prof ______________________________

Site no.: __________

Participant's name: _____________________________________

Participant's initials: __________ Participant ID no.: ______________

Participant's address: ____________________________________

MRN: ______ DOB: ___ / ___ / ___ Body weight: _______ Height: _______

Prescriber to write required investigational product dose and tick Visit No.:

One IP kit contains _____ vials, supplied in two different strengths, for subcutaneous injections

Visit No.

- ☐ Day 1 *(1 kit)*
- ☐ Week 1 *(3 kits)*
- ☐ Week 3 *(4 kits)*
- ☐ Week 6 *(6 kits)*
- ☐ Week 13 *(8 kits)*
- ☐ Week 20 *(7 kits)*
- ☐ Week 26 *(14 kits)*
- ☐ Week 39 *(14 kits)*
- ☐ Week 52 *(1 kits)*
- ☐ Unscheduled visit

Supply

- ☐ Investigational Product Name or Placebo *(___ mg/vial) or*
- ☐ Investigational Product Name or Placebo *(___ mg/vial)*

(Dose = ____ microgram/kg/day)

IP Kit No.: ____

(Attach IRT printout with assigned IP kits)

Directions for Use:

Reconstitute **one** vial with ____ **mL** Water for Injection and **Administer** ____ **mL** (= ____ mg) **daily** via subcutaneous injection at the same time each day. Use within ____ **hours** of preparation, as per protocol

____.

Doctor's name *(print)*: ______________________________

Pager/Phone No.: ______________________________

Signature: ______________________________

Date of prescription: ___ / ___ / ___

Clinical trial coordinator name: ______________________________

Contact details: ______________________________

CT PHARMACY USE ONLY

Date	Dispensed by	Checked by	Collected by and date

CT Service/Pharmacy Name: ______________________________

Address: ______________________________

Phone No.: ____________________ Fax No.: ____________________

Acknowledgements

I must start by thanking my family for accompanying me on this journey. The silver lining of writing this book during COVID-19 is the opportunity to create and experience long-lasting, intense memories and moments together. Thank you for your unwavering faith in me and for pushing me outside of my comfort zone by channelling my professional strengths throughout the journey.

Thank you, Diana, for your continuous and unparalleled love and guidance, ranging from thoughts, emotions, and impulses to techniques and mechanics. Thank you, Sam, for being the highly effective closer with unquivering thoughts, always at the right time, before the finale.

I want to express my most profound appreciation for Mr. T, who taught me the importance of wit, eat, sleep, and breathe, and spirit. Thank you for persistently making me conscious that if I can, I should. Thank you, Trae.

I am thankful to Westmead Children's Hospital principal investigators, research team members, researchers, sponsors/CROs, and their representatives I have collaborated with over the years and completed many CTs. Without them, my framework would not have been tested in practice and no lessons learned to write about.

I am thankful for the shoulders of giants before that, who opened the door, trusted me, and fought for my vision to improve on our delivery of paediatric patient-centred clinical care continuously. This book is for better future treatments for children.

Finally, but not least, I would like to thank my publisher, Scribe Media, for publishing *Evolving the Dinosaur* and all professionals who worked on the book, along with the ones who contributed from behind the scenes.

A special thank you to my publishing manager, Jericho, for always seamlessly illuminating the steps.

Thank you, Rachael, for the fantastic artwork. Thank you, Lisa, Will, and Holly, for editing my pharmaceutical "lingo" manuscript.

Notes

1 J. Lex, 'Why the Watchdog Won't Bite: U.S. Food and Drug Administration Challenges', *The Western Journal of Emergency Medicine*, 17, no. 6 (2016),:747–748, https://doi.org/10.5811/westjem.2016.9.32492.

2 E. Freye, 'Development of sensory information processing—the ontogenesis of opioid binding sites in nociceptive afferents and their significance in the clinical setting', *Acta Anaesthesiologica Scandinavica* 109 (Suppl.) (1996): 98-101, https://doi.org/10.1038/cipt.1988.127.

3 J. D. Momper, Y. Mulugeta, G. J. Burckart. 'Failed Pediatric Drug Development Trials', *Clinical Pharmacology & Therapeutics*, 98, no. 3 (2015): 245-251, https://doi.org/10.1002/cpt.142.

4 Ibid.

5 L. E. Kelly et al, 'Important Issues in the Justification of a Control Treatment in Paediatric Drug Trials. *Archives of Disease in Child*hood 101 (2016): 962–67.

6 P. D. Joseph et al, 'Completeness of Protocols for Clinical Trials in Children Submitted to Ethics Committees', *Journal of Paediatrics and Child Health*, 55, no. 3 (March 2019): 291–29, https://doi.org/10.1111/jpc.14189.

7 J. van den Anker, M. D. Reed, K. Allegaert, and G. L. Kearns, 'Developmental Changes in Pharmacokinetics and Pharmacodynamics', *The Journal of Clinical Pharmacology*, 58 (2018): S10–S25, https://doi.org/10.1002/jcph.1284.

8 K. Weimer et al. 'Placebo Effects in Children: A Review', *Pediatric Research* 74 (2013): 96–102, https://doi.org/10.1038/pr.2013.66.

9 D. Girard et al, 'How to Improve the Implementation of Academic Clinical Pediatric Trials Involving Drug Therapy? A Qualitative Study of Multiple Stakeholders', *PloS One*, 8, no. 5 (2013): e64516, https://doi.org/10.1371/journal.pone.0064516.

10 Elizabeth H. Follmer et al, 'Resolution, Relief, and Resignation: A Qualitative Study of Responses to Misfit at Work', *2018 Faculty Bibliography*, 22.

11 W. Arthur Jr., S. T. Bell, A. J. Villado, and D. Doverspike. 'The Use of Person–Organization Fit in Employment Decision Making: An Assessment of Its Criterion-Related Validity', *The Journal of Applied Psychology*, 91 (2006): 786–801.

12 J. R. Edwardset al, 'The Phenomenology of Fit: Linking the Person and Environment to the Subjective Experience of Person–Environment Fit', *The Journal of Applied Psychology*, 91 (2006): 802–827. B. Schneider. 'The people make the place,' *Personnel Psychology*, 40 (1987): 437–453.

13 Follmer et al, 'Resolution, Relief, and Resignation'. J. R. P. French, W. L. Rodgers, and S. Cobb, 'Adjustment as Person–Environment Fit,' in G. Coelho, D. Hamburg, and J. Adams (eds.) *Coping and Adaptation* (New York, NY: Basic Books, 1974), 316-333. R. V. Harrison. 'Person–Environment Fit and Job Stress,' in C. L. Cooper and R. Payne (eds.), *Stress at Work* (New York, NY: Wiley, 1978), 175–205.

14 K. Y. T. Yu, 'Affective Influences in Person–Environment Fit Theory: Exploring the Role of Affect as Both Cause and Outcome of P–E Fit, *The Journal of Applied Psychology*, 94 (2009): 1210–1226.

15 Robyn Keast, Michael Charles, and Piotr Modzelewski, 'The Cost of Collaboration: More than Budgeted for?', *The Power to Persuade*, April 10, 2017, http://www.powertopersuade.org.au/blog/the-cost-of-collaboration-more-than-budgeted-for/13/4/2017.

16 Girard et al, 'How to Improve the Implementation of Academic Clinical Pediatric Trials'.

17 H. O. La et al, 'Current Status and Future Directions for Clinical Trials Pharmacy', *Yakugaku Zasshi*. 131, no. 6 (2011): 969–75, https://doi.org//10.1248/yakushi.131.969.

18 J.I. Westbrook et al, 'Association of interruptions with an increased risk and severity of medication administration errors,' Archives of Internal Medicine, 170 no. 8 (2010): 683–690, https://doi.org/10.1001/archinternmed.2010.65.

19 G. S. Takata et al, 'Development, Testing, and Findings of a Pediatric-Focused Trigger Tool to Identify Medication-Related Harm in US Children's Hospitals', *Pediatrics*, 121 (2008): e927–3935, http://www.pediatrics.org/cgi/content/full/121/4/e927.

20 Karen Frush, Xuemei Luo, Paul Hutchinson, and Jennifer Higgins, 'Evaluation of a Method to Reduce Over-the-Counter Medication Dosing Error' *Archives of Pediatrics & Adolescent Medicine*, 158, no. 7 (July 2004): 620–4, https://doi.org/10.1001/archpedi.158.7.620.

21 S. El-Rachidi et al, 'Pharmacists and Pediatric Medication Adherence: Bridging the Gap', *Hospital Pharmacy* 52 (2017):124–31.

22 Roshana Gul, 'The Relationship between Reputation, Customer Satisfaction, Trust, and Loyalty', *Journal of Public Administration and Governance* 4 (2014): 368, https://doi.org/10.5296/jpag.v4i3.6678.

23 Rebecca McAvoy, 'The Quest To Improve Efficiency In Site Contract And Budget Negotiations' *Clinical Leader*, Industry Standard Research (ISR) report, Jan 13, 2020.

24 El-Rachidi et al, 'Pharmacists and Pediatric Medication Adherence.'

25 J. L. Bauman.,'Hero Clinical Pharmacists and the COVID-19 Pandemic: Overworked and Overlooked', *Journal of the American College of Clinical Pharmacy* 3 (2020): 721–22, https://doi.org/10.1002/jac5.1246.

Made in the USA
Middletown, DE
05 November 2026

36537970R10152

EVOLVING THE DINOSAUR